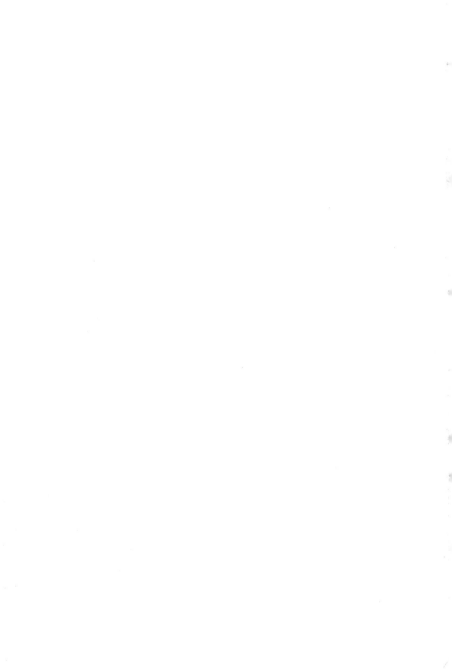

FULL
of
LIFE

Mom-to-Mom Tips I Wish Someone Had Told Me When I Was Pregnant

Nancy O'Dell

with Jessica Kaminsky

SSE

Simon Spotlight Entertainment

New York   London   Toronto   Sydney

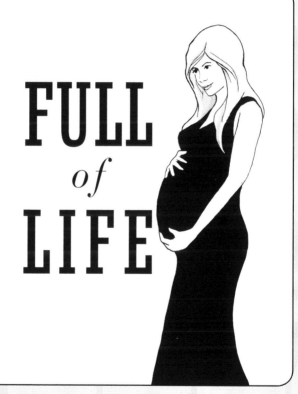

FULL *of* LIFE

I dedicate this book to the two women who have
made my life so full of love:
To my precious daughter, Ashby, who is the light of my life and has
brought me happiness beyond what I could have ever imagined.
I will always be there for you! Oh, how Mama loves you so!
To my precious mom, Betty, who passed away from
Lou Gehrig's disease in June 2008, three days before Ashby's
first birthday. You were the definition of an incredible mom.
You were always there for me and still are, I know, as my angel.

Simon Spotlight Entertainment
A Division of Simon & Schuster, Inc.
1230 Avenue of the Americas
New York, NY 10020

First Simon Spotlight Entertainment hardcover edition April 2009

SIMON SPOTLIGHT ENTERTAINMENT and colophon are trademarks
of Simon & Schuster, Inc.

For information about special discounts for bulk purchases,
please contact Simon & Schuster Special Sales at 1-866-506-1949 or
business@simonandschuster.com.

The Simon & Schuster Speakers Bureau can bring authors to your live event.
For more information or to book an event contact the Simon & Schuster
Speakers Bureau at 1-866-248-3049 or visit our website at www.simonspeakers.com.

Designed by Nancy Singer; illustrations copyright © 2009 by Sarah Jane Wright

Manufactured in the United States of America

10 9 8 7 6 5 4 3 2 1

Library of Congress Cataloging-in-Publication Data is available.

ISBN   978-1-4391-2391-1

CONTENTS

INTRODUCTION

I was seven months pregnant when my friends and co-workers from *Access Hollywood* threw me a baby shower brunch. At that point I knew I was having a girl—little Miss Ashby Grace would soon arrive on the scene, on June 11, 2007—which meant that the restaurant was covered in pink balloons and confetti. The tables were decorated with darling little mesh bunny rabbits filled with jellybeans. And then there was the dessert: my pals had made a cake out of donuts for me. Early in my pregnancy, I had developed an insane craving for donuts. And they couldn't be just any kind of donut. They had to be plain glazed, heated for *exactly* fifteen seconds in the microwave. I had it down to a science. And everyone at *Access* knew it.

But what I didn't have down to a science was all of the things that happen during pregnancy, birth, and those first few days home with a new baby. So after we finished opening gifts at the shower, we played a game where people wrote down on slips of paper little bits of advice and words of wisdom about what I could expect during the rest of my pregnancy, in the delivery room, and once Ashby was born. The tips were great! One friend told me, "Preregister at the hospital." *Huh? You can preregister for the baby's birth before you even go into labor? How is that possible?* Well, it turns out that yes, you can, and this prevents you from having to worry about all that paperwork when you're in labor, having contractions, and about to add a new member to the family. Instead, you can focus on what you came to do: have the baby!

Another friend wrote, "Don't be surprised if you have headlights (you know, hard nipples) during your pregnancy." No kidding! I had already found that one out the hard way (no pun intended). But I wish I had known about it before I arrived on the set of *Grey's Anatomy* to conduct an interview, looking like I was a little too happy to see Doctors McDreamy and McSteamy.

These suggestions made me realize that there are so many unexpected, sometimes terrifying, sometimes gross things that happen during pregnancy that just aren't talked about enough. Where were all of these reassuring tips and kernels of wisdom when I first found out that I was going to become a mom? Yes, countless books have been written on the subject of pregnancy. But as I quickly discovered, there are many things that are *not* covered in the pregnancy books—at least, not in the ones I read, and I read a lot of them. Like, what about the time my chest broke out in little red dots—what on earth was that? I completely panicked! Did I have the measles? The mumps? Chicken pox? My blood pressure shot up sky high as I wondered what was wrong with me and how it was affecting my baby. Well, after a visit with my doctor (whom I think is great and who was always so reassuring), I was told that what I was experiencing was absolutely nothing to be alarmed about. In fact, the dots I'd developed on my chest were completely normal during pregnancy, and they would go away after I had the baby. (I swear my makeup artist had to become a magician during my pregnancy.) You can turn to pages 75–76 to read the medical explanation he gave me, but the bottom line is I could've had one less panic attack if any of the books I'd bought had mentioned that a red-dotted chest was par for the course during pregnancy for some women.

I'm an information junkie. The reporter in me never rests. So from the moment my husband, Keith, and I set about trying to get pregnant, I had many questions, starting with *how long does it take to get pregnant?* Answer: it takes an average of six months to conceive. Well, phew. What a relief to know that you haven't flunked the fertility test if you don't get pregnant on the first try. And once it was confirmed that I was officially pregnant, I was constantly on the computer, looking up *everything*. My doctor and I spoke so often we were practically on a first-name basis with each other. And I found myself asking all of my friends with kids a zillion and one questions, only to discover that your friends don't always remember to tell you half of the things that happened to them during their pregnancies.

I also found that some of the books that are available are helpful but hard to navigate, especially the ones with a forty-page index. Plus, I felt that a lot of the things that you experience during your pregnancy that aren't harmful to you or your baby (such as red dots on your chest) aren't even mentioned in these books. But guess what? If it happens to you and you don't know it's not harmful . . . it's *scary*! That is why I wanted to share in a simple, fun, straightforward book all of those crazy, unexpected, sometimes disgusting, sometimes hilarious things that happened to me during my pregnancy. I took notes throughout my pregnancy so I would have a record of what I was experiencing (again, the reporter in me never rests), and now I'm passing them on to you in hopes that you won't be too surprised when some of these things happen to you.

P.S. While I wrote this introduction, my daughter, who was sleeping next to me, opened her eyes, smiled at

Mama, crawled onto my chest to cuddle with me, then fell back to sleep. My heart practically melted. So no matter how challenging pregnancy can be, trust me . . . it's all worth it!

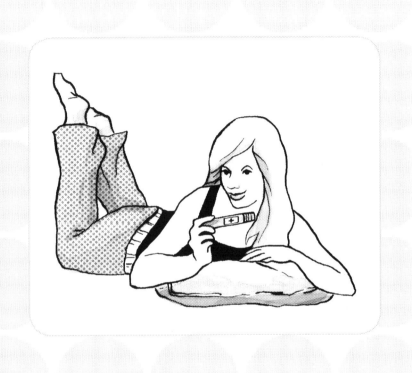

PRE-CONCEPTION

My husband, Keith, and I always knew we wanted to have kids. So after we had been married for a while, we wanted to expand our family. Keith already had two beautiful boys—Tyler and Carson, whom I adore—from his first marriage; they have their mom, and I'm their "Nommy," their Nancy mommy. But ever since I was young, I always knew I wanted to have a baby of my own. So there I was. I had met the man of my dreams, we had gotten married, I was beyond happy, and it felt like all the pieces were falling into place. *So, let's do it,* I thought. *Let's have a baby!*

The first thing I did after Keith and I decided to try to get pregnant was make an appointment with my gynecologist. "What do we need to do?" I asked. "Well," he said, laughing, "you need to have intercourse. And a lot of it." Yeah. I knew that one. But all kidding aside, I had questions . . . many questions.

The Numbers Game

I asked my doctor, "How long does it take for women to conceive?" The answer: Typical fertile couples (and I already knew Keith had swimmers) have a 20 percent chance of becoming pregnant with each cycle and an 85 percent chance of becoming pregnant within one year. It's true that a year is a long time, and can feel much longer when you're waiting for that little line to appear on a pregnancy test. But those odds seemed pretty good to me.

Peak Time

During that first visit, I also learned from my doctor when women are most fertile. In most cases, you're at peak fertility one to two days before ovulation and up to twenty-four hours after. The doctor explained that this had to do with the fact that while sperm cells can live two to three days inside of you, an egg survives for only twenty-four hours. Of course, as the doctor told me these things, I was taking meticulous mental notes. Pregnancy, or at least getting pregnant, suddenly seemed much more complicated than I'd initially thought. And to top it off, every celebrity I was covering for *Access Hollywood* seemed to be pregnant or had just given birth—Angelina, Britney, Katie Holmes, Gwyneth Paltrow, Mariska Hargitay. I could feel the pressure mounting.

Prep Work

One thing that didn't surprise me during my visit to the ob-gyn was when my doctor prescribed a prenatal vitamin for me. As a spokesperson for the March of Dimes, I know how important it is for all women who are even considering getting pregnant to take a prenatal vitamin. Here's why: Prenatal vitamins are high in folic acid, which can prevent birth defects of the brain and spinal cord (such as spina bifida). Not to mention, a prenatal vitamin helps provide extra amounts of iron and calcium. While a vitamin isn't a substitute for a healthy diet, it goes a long way toward making sure that women receive sufficient levels of the right minerals to create a healthy child.

Charting Ovulation

Back to the business of getting pregnant: we needed to have sex and we needed to have a lot of it. Doctor's orders! My husband wasn't complaining. But after weeks of diligently trying, when, at the end of the month, I'd get my period, I couldn't help but feel vaguely disappointed. Common sense told me there was nothing to be concerned about. I had read the websites and knew the statistics. And yet, I still felt defeated.

Several months into actively trying to put a bun in the oven, I decided to get serious. I was determined to address whatever was happening (or *not* happening) head on. So I began to chart my menstrual cycle meticulously. I bought an ovulation calculator, those pee sticks that can tell you when you're ovulating; a basal body thermometer to chart my fertility; and—I kid you not—a "fertility scope" (a mini-microscope type of device that you put on your tongue), which supposedly can detect whether you are ovulating based on the composition of your saliva. If there was a product on the market that could help me conceive, chances are I had it. Meanwhile, whenever my husband and I went out, we'd see pregnant women *everywhere*. And I swear it felt as if every other story I read for *Access* was about the "Hollywood Baby Boom." It was starting to feel personal. Why wasn't I pregnant?

The Buddy System

If you're feeling discouraged, my advice is: find a friend and buddy up. It helps to have sisterly support in your baby-making efforts, as well as someone to make you feel as if you're not alone in your quest to get pregnant. This really helped me. By happy coincidence, my very close childhood friend Abby was also trying to conceive at the same time. She and I would compare notes and share tips. That way, when another month rolled by and neither of us had a positive EPT stick to show for ourselves, we'd lift each other up with words of encouragement. "It'll happen next month. You'll see."

Abby had become my pregnancy partner in crime. The funny thing is that when I learned I was pregnant, I sat down at the computer to e-mail her my good news, only to discover an e-mail from her: she was pregnant, too! So, you see, the buddy system can work. Find a friend and partner up. Just be sure to pick someone with whom you can be open and honest. And if you don't have a buddy in your circle of friends who is trying to get pregnant, there are many pregnancy websites with forums where women can share their experiences.

DOUBLE THE FUN

If you wind up pregnant at the same time as a friend, consider a joint shower. My high school friends, Lane and Sonja, came up with this idea for me and Abby. It was like a mini high school reunion!

The Sex-a-thon

While we were trying to conceive, I spoke to another one of my childhood friends, Jan. I was telling her about how Keith and I had been trying and it wasn't working, and she stopped me midsentence and said, "I'll totally tell you how to get pregnant." And there, sitting on the beach in our hometown of Myrtle Beach, South Carolina, with both of our husbands next to us, Jan shared her method. She leaned in and said, "So here's what you have to do: have sex ten days in a row." Keith nodded with a big grin. Jan continued. "You have to have sex five days before your suspected ovulation date and five days after. And you have to do it at approximately the same time every day." Basically, it's like a sex-a-thon. The key, Jan explained, was committing to the rules. Keith and I looked at each other. We were in. So we followed the "ten days in a row" method. It didn't always result in our most romantic nights, but we stuck to the schedule. And you know what? It worked!

Just Relax

Looking back—and this is an important note—even though we followed the ten-day method, at the time I really didn't think I was going to get pregnant. I had started to believe we'd have to turn to science, which somehow took the pressure off and helped me to relax. The next thing I knew . . . BOOM! I was pregnant. We ended up conceiving 100 percent naturally. (Thank you, sex-a-thon!) I really believe it's because we were finally able to relax. So, try to relax! I know it's not easy, but I think it truly helps.

Hey, Lady! Turn Down Those Headlights

I knew that nausea, tender boobs, and exhaustion were possible signs of pregnancy. But I had *never* heard anything about hard nipples. It wasn't in any of my books, and none of my friends had mentioned they'd experienced it, which left me to discover this one on my own. Apparently, the elevation of the tiny glands around the nipple is one indication of pregnancy. However, I didn't know this when Keith and I were keeping our fingers crossed that we'd gotten pregnant. So, basically, I spent an entire week with my headlights on high.

The first time I noticed my extroverted nipples was in the shower. *Why were they hard?* I wondered. The water wasn't cold. And I certainly wasn't aroused at 6:00 A.M. Then I noticed them again when I was getting dressed for *Access.* I walked into Wardrobe, convinced they'd given me the wrong bra. "Where's the thicker bra? You know, the one I usually wear?" Of course, everyone thought I was crazy. "Nancy, this *is* the bra you always wear." And when I got home, my husband took one look at my high beams and figured his wife was in the mood. Little did we know that I had a bun cooking in the oven.

Are You Positive?

Home pregnancy tests have become so advanced that you can pee on a stick five days before you get your period and learn if you're with child. Which is exactly what I did. I couldn't wait until the first day of my missed period—I needed to know as soon as possible.

9

So I peed on the stick and waited for the results. I tried to be Zen about it, but I swear, three minutes have never felt longer. When the time was up, I took a deep breath, turned the stick over, and there, smack dab in the middle of my EPT stick, was a very faint line. I called Keith in and said, "Am I crazy or is there a line there?" Keith thought he saw something, but he wasn't sure. I took two more tests—same faint line results, but we both agreed that it looked like something was there. What it meant, if anything, was another story. I had to go to work, so I stuffed the remains of my various home pregnancy tests in my purse and ran out the door.

I was so excited I called my sister, Karen, and my mom with the "Guess what? I think I might be pregnant" news. My sister was cautiously optimistic and said, "I think *maybe* that's good news that you *think* you *might* be pregnant." I quizzed her on whether she thought the faint line meant I was pregnant, but she didn't know. Finally, I called my doctor for him to weigh in on what an almost-maybe-possibly line on a pregnancy test meant. He explained that the way the tests work is by detecting the presence of the pregnancy hormone hCG (human chorionic gonadotropin) in the urine. So even though the line was faint, there was a good darn chance it meant I was pregnant! My doctor then told me to take the test again in the morning, when the presence of the pregnancy hormone would be even stronger. Turns out that that hormone (the one that produces a positive result) doubles itself every twenty-four hours. He suspected I would have a much darker line the next day.

I woke up at 5:00 A.M. to pee on a stick. My doctor was right. There was no question—the line was dark. I was definitely pregnant!

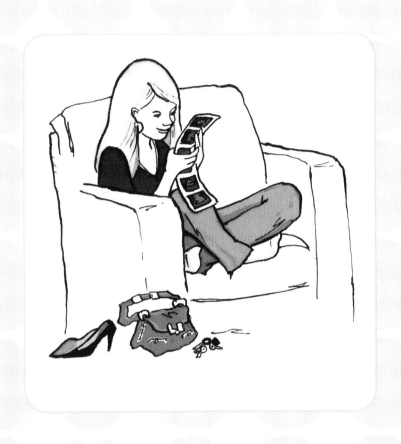

FIRST TRIMESTER

The first trimester (zero to fourteen weeks) is filled with so many emotions. Keith and I were beyond thrilled. We were pregnant, by golly! But we weren't ready to shout the news from the rooftops yet.

First off, I wanted to keep the circle of people who knew about my pregnancy limited to family and a few close friends for a while. Most pregnant women do, since the chance of a miscarriage is greatest in the first twelve weeks. I had gotten news from my doctor that the hormone levels from my formal pregnancy blood test were strong—a good sign your pregnancy will stick—but again, you never know.

Second, there was work. I definitely wanted to wait until I was officially out of the first trimester before I shared the news with my co-workers at *Access Hollywood*. But let's be honest, by the time I did spill the beans, you'd have to have been blind not to know. I'll never forget when my co-host and friend, Billy Bush, casually leaned over when I was nine weeks pregnant and said, "I love my wife and I don't want to be rude, but you appear a tad top-heavy . . . Hello! Either you've upgraded or you're pregnant." I was busted. I looked at him and said, "Billy, your microphone is on!" I felt like I had a spotlight shining down on me at that moment. I actually did have a spotlight on me, as we were taping the show, but this one felt like a searchlight! *Did everybody else in the studio now suspect that I was pregnant as well?* I wondered. I tried to play it off. "Oh, stop it. That's ridiculous!" But just like the scene in *Knocked Up* where Katherine Heigl tries to suck in her baby belly, pretty much *everyone* knew I was pregnant. I just didn't know they knew!

There were my wardrobe stylists, Daniel and Nicole. These people see me naked as often as, maybe even more than, my husband. So why I thought they wouldn't notice my ever-expanding belly I have no clue. I guess for the first time ever in my Hollywood life, I actually hoped they thought I was just gaining weight. But when my pants wouldn't button *again,* Daniel gave me a knowing look. I turned to him and said, "You think I'm pregnant, too, don't you?" He looked me up and down and said, "Nanny-O, I know you're pregnant, but you feel free to tell me when you're ready." I laughed and tried to change the subject. But seriously, was it that obvious?

The same thing happened with my makeup artist, Karen. She's in charge of making me look glamorous and camera-ready every day, and this task includes applying foundation to my chest. One day she started drumming on my boobs with her makeup brush. I looked at her and said, "Karen, what are you doing?" She smiled and said, "Your boobs are just so bouncy." "You think I'm pregnant, huh?" I was starting to sound like a broken record. Karen looked me in the eye and said, "I knew a month ago, but you feel free to tell me when you're ready." The truth was, I couldn't wait to share the news. I just wasn't ready yet, since I hadn't reached the end of my first trimester.

On a Serious Note

One of the reasons I wasn't quite ready to tell people I was expecting is that before I got pregnant with Ashby I had a miscarriage. I've never mentioned this publicly until now, but I think it's important to talk about, especially since my doctor told me just how frequently miscarriages can occur. I had no idea that approximately one in four pregnancies end in miscarriage, with some estimates as high as one in three.

When I went to my doctor's office for an examination after miscarrying, I sat in the exam room crying. The nurse asked why I was so sad. I said, "I just had a miscarriage and I so wanted to be pregnant." She replied, as if it were no big deal, "Oh, don't worry. You'll get pregnant again. It's a good sign that you were able to conceive." With the knowledge I have now, I realize the nurse was only trying to be comforting because she knew the statistics. But my miscarriage felt like a very big deal to me—I was only seven weeks pregnant when I miscarried, but it was a loss, and I certainly was mourning.

It would have been so much easier if the weight of silence didn't hang over the subject. Later, when I told several of my friends about my miscarriage, I was surprised to learn that many of them had gone through the same thing. One told me, "Oh, yeah. I had a miscarriage." Another friend said, "I had three." So even though the subject had gone virtually unmentioned throughout my experience, it was comforting to know I wasn't alone. Plus, before I knew the statistics, I worried that something was wrong with me. My doctor assured me this was not the case and that I would get pregnant again. And of course, you know where the story goes from there . . . I did get pregnant again, with my precious little Ashby.

Overwhelming Undergarments

One of the most surprising aspects of the first trimester was how much my body changed in a few short weeks. I think pretty much everybody knows that when you're pregnant your boobs get bigger. But none of the books mention how you get *so* big, *so* quickly. Within a matter of weeks, I went from a small C to a busty D. It was borderline pornographic.

Anyway, no surprise, none of my bras fit me anymore. I had to go shopping, so I grabbed my sister-in-law, Jenny, and we headed to the mall. Because I'm on TV and I hadn't officially announced my pregnancy, I didn't want to say anything to the saleslady in the lingerie department. But as I stood flipping through the rack, I had no clue what size I had become. Jenny couldn't tell through my bulky top, so we slipped into the dressing room. I raised my shirt, and Jenny exclaimed, "Holy moly, Nancy! You're gigantic! You're gonna have to ask the saleslady for help, because I can't even begin to guess your size." Finally, I broke down, and turned to the woman who worked at the store and said, "Please don't say anything to anyone, but I'm eight weeks pregnant and I'm *huge*! Can you please help me?" It was crazy to think that some of my oldest friends didn't know I was expecting, but there I was, in a random store, sharing my news with a complete stranger. But it was for a good cause. The girls (my boobs) needed help. And they needed it fast.

Sexy Lingerie

One thing I discovered while I was buying new bras is that there's *no* sexy lingerie for pregnant ladies. (Hmm . . . possible business idea? Maybe.) I searched the lingerie store high and low for something that would accommodate my growing baby bump, but still make me look and feel sexy. Either the clothes fit on the top and looked like a burhka on the bottom, or they were way too tight and uncomfortable all over.

So here's my tip: Buy a "tap pant set." Basically, that's a fitted top that comes with matching shorts, but the top and pants are sold separately. This way, you can buy the top so that it's big enough for your boobs, and then you can get a smaller size for the bottom and wear the shorts below the belly. It's a very cute look. Your mate will be pleased, I promise.

Tender Is the Night

For the first time in my life I had huge knockers. And they were all mine for nine whole months. Time to have a little fun with them, right? Wrong! Tender doesn't even begin to describe the way my boobs felt. First of all, they were hot. Temperature hot, that is. They felt like you could fry an egg on them. Second, if my husband so much as brushed past them, they'd hurt. One time Keith completely forgot and gave them a good old squeeze. I jumped so high you would've thought I had been mugged. But there is a silver lining: after the first trimester, the tenderness does die down. The tenderness never totally went away, but if properly handled, my breasts could be touched. So if your mate is a boob man, he doesn't have to give up his favorite body part completely for the duration of the pregnancy. Just let him know what feels good and what doesn't, and remind him that there's a rainbow at the end of the first trimester.

Mom's Version of Teething Pain

Well, if it isn't one thing, then it's another. First I noticed that my boobs were sensitive. Next, it was my gums. When they first started hurting I thought that it must have been a side effect of the spicy food I had for lunch. But after a few days of eating mild foods, my gums *still* hurt. That's when I learned that swollen gums are common during pregnancy. Great! Add that to the list of indignities. The inflammation of the gums is called "pregnancy gingivitis" and is caused by the hormonal changes that increase the blood flow to the gum tissue, so your gums become sensitive and swollen.

Was it going to be this painful for my entire pregnancy? Or was this just a temporary trimester thing? My dentist told me that your gums usually return to normal after the delivery of your baby. (Ugh. I was only in my first trimester.) The good news was he had a few tips on how to ease the pain. He recommended that I switch to a softer toothbrush, use a saltwater rinse daily, and floss at least once a day. I followed his orders, and my gums did start to feel better.

More Than Skin Deep

The week after I found out I was pregnant, I was on the set of the TV show *Nip/Tuck* when it occurred to me I should be careful about what I put on my skin now that

I had a baby on board. Billy and I were there to interview the cast for an episode set in the future. The actors had been aged via the magic of professional makeup, and the *Nip/Tuck* producers thought it might be fun for Billy and me to conduct our interviews made up as old folks. I thought it would be fun too . . . *until* the makeup artist brought out a tub of some thick, awful-looking sticky paste. She wanted to slather it on my face in order to glue the "old people" prosthetics on. Panic! *If she puts this on my skin,* I wondered, *could it be absorbed into my body and affect the baby?* Fortunately, I had a laptop within arm's reach and was able to do some research via the Internet. My suspicions were confirmed. According to various websites, some topical ingredients *are* absorbed into the bloodstream, and once an ingredient entered my bloodstream it could enter the baby's circulation, so I needed to be extra careful about staying away from ingredients with scientific links to birth defects.

I *knew* I had to say something, but I hadn't yet told anyone I was pregnant, as it was so early. I scribbled a note on a sheet of paper for the makeup artist that read: *I am pregnant, but I haven't told anyone yet. I don't want to put the sticky stuff on my face for fear it might be absorbed into my body.* The irony didn't escape me that yet another person I had just met had learned my news before even some of my closest friends. But, the makeup artist was great. She smiled at me and cleverly said out loud, "Nancy, I can tell by looking at your skin that it is sensitive. I'm going to use a different application mix for you than we are using on Billy. It is water-based and all natural. Your prosthetics won't last as long as Billy's, but I think it will be better for your feminine skin." Mission accomplished.

Later that day, I called my ob-gyn and my dermatologist, who confirmed that there are a handful of ingredients considered potentially harmful to a growing baby, and that I should always read labels before putting anything on my body. They specifically mentioned retinoids, salicylic acid, and benzoyl peroxide as products to avoid while pregnant. My suggestion to any expectant mom is to take all of your lotions and potions to your doctor, have them read the labels, and tell you specifically which of your products are safe to continuing using. I did this, and it made me feel much better!

COSMETIC CONUNDRUMS

Be aware, even some makeup products include retinoids and salicylic acid. My dermatologist told me if I wanted to be super careful to try some of the minerals-only makeup lines or those marked "noncomedogenic" or "nonacnegenic."

Sun Spots

After I became pregnant, I noticed that I started getting brown spots on my face. Yes, pregnant women are susceptible to splotchy pigmentation. The brown spots are caused by hormones and sun exposure, and are aggravated by the sun. So did that mean I could no longer enjoy a day in the sun? Not the case. Titanium dioxide and zinc oxide are powerful sunscreens and do not penetrate the skin.

The Nose Knows

While I was having hardly any morning sickness (and I was so grateful for that), I was extremely sensitive to odors. Trust me, prepare yourself: your nose becomes like a hound dog's. My doctor explained that I could blame hormones for this. Ah, those pesky little hormones! Apparently, estrogen can make every little scent that comes your way seem like an all-out attack on your nostrils. For instance, leftovers could not go in the fridge. They had to be disposed of right after the meal. The garbage had to be taken out immediately. And don't even get me started on cologne. Keith couldn't wear it, and I couldn't be near it. But the worst of all my pregnancy-related aversions was my newfound distaste for chicken. I couldn't stand the smell of it. In fact, I couldn't even be in the same room with it!

Label Snob

Everyone's heard stories about pregnant women and their crazy cravings: ice cream and pickles. Ham sandwiches in the middle of the night. Giant slabs of barely cooked meat. So, comparatively, my first craving was relatively tame: I loved animal crackers. I kept a stash at home and a stash at work. I didn't need to eat them all the time. But when I wanted them, man oh man, get out of my way. The unusual thing I discovered about my craving was that it was *brand-specific*! I didn't like just any animal crackers. They had to be Nabisco, in the rectangular box with the circus animals on the outside and that cute little string handle. I once sent Keith out for a box of animal crackers, only to send him right back out again when he returned with another brand of animal crackers. How could he? What was he thinking? Moral of the story: Be aware that your cravings may be very specific. And no one should stand in the way of your enjoying them.

One-day Cravings

Before you head to Costco and load up on an industrial-size jug of olives, my advice is first try eating one normal-size jar. Because I found that some cravings last for only *one* day. It's true. I was about three months pregnant with Ashby when I suddenly started having a *major* craving for baked beans. I thought if I didn't have a plate of baked beans, I would just die. So I ran off the set of *Access Hollywood,* drove to the grocery store, and bought fifteen cans of baked beans. Then I went back to the office, ate one can, satisfied my craving, and never had it again. The only problem was that I had fourteen cans left, so

Keith and I wound up having a barbecue just so we could get rid of them.

Got Milk?

In the middle of my first trimester I noticed that my body was sending me messages in the form of cravings. So I stopped to listen. And for the first time, in a *really* long time, I found myself wanting milk. And I'm not talking about just a splash of milk. Oh, no. I was craving giant glasses of cold milk, filled to the brim. And sometimes one glass just wasn't enough. Later, I learned that at that stage of my pregnancy, Ashby's teeth were forming. In other words, my body wanted calcium to help Ashby's teeth develop. So you never know when your body will do the talking to tell you what you need. Just be sure to listen.

The Pregnancy Timetable (i.e., determining how far along you really are)

After it was confirmed I was pregnant, I remember the doctor telling me that I was four weeks along. Four weeks? But I had ovulated only two weeks before! How did my doctor get that number?

This is where things get complicated. We have always heard that women are pregnant for nine months (i.e., thirty-six weeks). And yet the average pregnancy lasts for forty weeks. So how is pregnancy *really* calculated? Well,

Scaling the First Trimester

One of the things you are asked to do every time you visit your doctor during pregnancy is to step on a scale. I was a little leery of getting weighed during my eight-week visit because I had been shopping the day before and noticed that I had gone up a full clothing size. My suspicions were confirmed when the scale showed I had gained eight pounds. I had read that the American College of Obstetricians and Gynecologists recommends a weight gain of three to five pounds in the first trimester, and a weight gain of twenty-five to thirty-seven pounds during the whole pregnancy for women who were an average weight before pregnancy. When my doctor saw the numbers, he told me not to diet, but just to be aware of what I was eating and to make sure it was healthy food. I told him I had already been making a conscious effort to eat well. (To this day, I swear those extra pounds were due to my rapidly expanding boobs.) My doctor explained that gaining too much weight during pregnancy can lead to gestational diabetes, which is bad for both the mother and the unborn baby. Since I was eating healthfully, he suspected my weight gain would level off in the second trimester, and it did.

your doctor begins counting from the first day of your last period. In other words, the two weeks before you conceived are considered part of your pregnancy. It's almost like your doctor is counting those two weeks based on spermicidal intent. In fact, the doctor considers the prep your body goes through to make a comfy home for the egg as part of the pregnancy. It's very confusing.

So let's review: A typical pregnancy lasts for forty weeks. The doctor counts the two weeks before you conceive, adds nine months, and then gets the final two weeks by adding together all of the extra days of the month (the twenty-ninth, thirtieth, thirty-first). Thus, bringing your pregnancy to a grand total of ten months. Not nine months, which is what all new moms expect.

PREGNANCY AS A MATH EQUATION

If pregnancy were a math equation, it would look something like this:

```
    2     weeks (nest prep)
+  36     weeks (9 months x 4 weeks)
+   2     weeks (all those extra days of the month)
   ──
=  40     weeks
```

Track Your Period . . . Period!

Once you decide to try to get pregnant it *really* helps to keep track of your menstrual cycle. Your due date is calculated using a formula, based on your period. One way to calculate is to add seven days to the first day of your last period. Then subtract three months, and add one year. Yes, it sounds tricky. But don't worry, your doctor will do the calculation, not you.

I had been recording the dates of my menstrual cycle so meticulously, to best predict when I was ovulating, that my due date calculation was almost dead on. Ashby was born one day after her projected due date. So I strongly recommend marking the days of your period on a calendar—it'll help your doctor and you to plan ahead. If you haven't marked down the days of your period, try to figure it out now, while it's still fresh in your mind.

It's a Miracle

Music has always put a time stamp on touchstone moments in my life. So it's not surprising that when I was pregnant I had an album I listened to over and over again: Celine Dion's *Miracle.* I've always been a huge fan of Celine's voice, and all of the songs on this CD are about children (the "miracle" of life). Each song is as beautiful as the next, and each pulls at the heartstrings as much as the next. And boy, did Keith know it. He had the CD loaded in his car and whenever I was in the car with him, he would slyly put it on just to see how long it would take me to tear up. I kid you not, I would start crying in 10.2 seconds. And to this day, listening to that CD brings back all the amazing feelings and emotions I had during that special time in my life.

So be aware that while you're pregnant you will have a sensitivity to *anything* regarding children. Just hearing someone sing about the joys of being a parent made me tear up.

Our First Ultrasound

Six weeks into my pregnancy, we got to see little Miss Ashby for the first time (although, of course, we didn't know if she was a "miss" or a "mister" at that point). The baby looked like a fuzzy dot on the monitor, but she was truly amazing. I couldn't believe a tiny person, whom I could *see,* was growing inside my body. All I can say is thank God the doctor wasn't playing any Celine Dion. I was already a puddle of emotion.

I recommend that you start your baby scrapbook on the day of your first ultrasound, the first time you see your little one. Granted, it may just look like a dot on the page, but that's your baby! You will have many more ultrasounds in the weeks to come, and it's so much fun to see the progression of life. So on every visit, ask for a copy of the ultrasound as a souvenir. I asked for three copies each time—one for us and a copy to send to each set of grandparents. My mom made a look-book out of just the ultrasounds, and it is so incredible to look at it now.

To this day, I still carry around in my wallet a copy of that first ultrasound of Ashby, which reads, "Hello," next to the fuzzy dot that was my daughter. And if I'm having a bad day, I pull it out and am reminded that this is what makes life worth living!

BE STILL, MY BEATING HEART

We weren't sure if we'd be able to hear the baby's heartbeat during our sixth-week visit. In fact, I had read that usually you are not able to hear the heartbeat until the tenth week. But our sixth-week appointment was October 16, my mom's birthday, and I had this sixth sense that we would hear it. And, guess what? We did! It was strong and steady, and one of the happiest moments of my pregnancy.

Your Pregnancy Scrapbook

There will be so many happy moments during your pregnancy and I highly recommend making a pregnancy scrapbook to preserve those memories. I am a huge scrapbooker. I keep pretty much *everything* that has to do with *anything* in our lives.

A pregnancy scrapbook includes everything from the moment you found out you were pregnant to the day you brought the baby home. You will treasure it for years to come. You can even save it and give it to your son or daughter as a present when they're expecting!

To start, buy an empty scrapbook and pages. I always use acid-free paper, as it will not deteriorate over time the way regular paper will; it is easy to find at a craft store or via the Internet. Then, simply start collecting items you want to add to the scrapbook. Here are a few suggestions:

Photos

* Your positive EPT (This can be the first photo in your scrapbook!)
* You and your mate the day you saw your positive pregnancy test
* Ultrasound photos—Ultrasounds are printed on a very thin paper, which deteriorates over time. Therefore, I made copies of mine on thick, good-quality photo paper and then laminated them. I recommend you do the same to make them last throughout the years.
* Baby shower shots—photos of the hostesses, guests, gifts, games, decorations, and even food (I have the cutest pictures of the donut cake from my baby shower, and what fun memories that photo brings back of my cravings!)

- The nursery, before and after
- Close-ups of the nursery furniture and bedding
- Siblings and grandparents with your expanding belly
- Belly shots at regular intervals (from the side, of course!)
- Meaningful occasions, to document what you were doing as the pregnancy progressed (I took a picture with every celebrity I interviewed during my pregnancy. I thought Ashby might get a kick out of knowing she had been introduced to the likes of Madonna, Leonardo DiCaprio, Richard Gere, Will Smith, Halle Berry, George Clooney, Celine Dion, Robin Williams, and other well-known people while she was in my tummy.)
- Labor and delivery shots
- Coming-home-from-the-hospital photos
- Baby's first house

Things to Write About

- How you felt when you found out you were pregnant
- How you told others
- The reactions of siblings, your parents, friends
- Your feelings when you found out the baby's gender
- Your cravings
- Your dreams
- Songs you listened to while pregnant
- Baby names you considered

Things to Record

* Your weight at regular intervals
* The measurement of your belly at regular intervals
* The cost of nursery items (for your child to compare costs when he or she has a baby)

Memorabilia

You can purchase clear plastic envelopes that are made for displaying memorabilia in scrapbooks. I recommend including:

* Shower invitations
* Advice from your girlfriends (ask them to record their tips at the shower, as I did)
* Swatches of fabric from nursery bedding or drapery
* Nursery paint color samples

Pages from Your Calendar

I chart everything in my Day-Timer. It is so interesting now to pull out the pages from when I was pregnant and see what I was doing when Ashby was developing. I think she will enjoy reading it when she is pregnant.

A Family Tree

Show your baby from whom he or she is descended.

What to Expect When You Get Your First Ultrasound

The first time we went to the doctor after finding out we were pregnant, he came in to the examination room and told us that we were going to do an ultrasound. Great, I thought, and started to lift my gown, expecting that the technician would cover my belly with some sort of gel and then use that rolling-ball apparatus on my tummy, just like in the movies. But the doctor stopped me and said, "Actually, we'll be doing the ultrasound vaginally." *What?* He pulled out a long wand that looked *a lot* like a vibrator and, to make matters even stranger, started fitting it with a condom. I sat up straight. "You're going to do *what* with *what*?" I asked. Yikes!

The doctor explained that we'd be doing a "transvaginal" ultrasound, which is used early in a pregnancy because it's a more precise way of seeing and hearing the baby in the first weeks. (This is how we were able to hear little Ashby's heartbeat so early.) The science behind the rolling-ball and the wand ultrasounds is the same: the instrument records the echoes of sound waves as they bounce off the baby, which then translates into a picture for you to see on the monitor. But here's the bottom line, ladies: don't be alarmed when your gynecologist whips out what appears to be a giant plastic penis. And note: the condom is used to keep the device sterile, not because the wand could get you pregnant.

Loose Lips

At seven weeks, Keith and I went to get our second scheduled ultrasound. Already I was addicted. I just loved being able to see our little baby on the screen and watch how she'd grown. And I couldn't believe that in one short week, our baby had doubled in size and was now measuring about half an inch. (Or, to put it another way, she was the size of a blueberry.)

At that point, we still didn't know if Ashby was a guy or a gal. Keith and I were both staring at the monitor, in a state of awe and wonderment, when all of a sudden the ultrasound technician blurted out, "I think you're having a boy!" We had never told the technician that we wanted to know the sex of the baby! Lesson one: Tell *everyone* in your doctor's office whether you want to know your baby's sex. Lesson two: *All* babies look like boys in the beginning.

Oh, and that "penis" the Chatty Cathy technician had pointed out on the ultrasound monitor was in fact the baby's tail. Yes, a baby has a tail in the very beginning stages of pregnancy, which is just an extension of their tailbone. But don't worry, the tail disappears within a few weeks— just around the time you will be able to see if you're having a boy or a girl!

CVS Is Not Just a Drugstore

CVS, or chorionic villus sampling, is a test used to detect chromosomal abnormalities early in pregnancy.

36

Think of it as an early amnio. The procedure involves a needle, which is used to collect a tiny sample of the placental tissue from the uterus. The test feels a little more intense than a pap smear, and the procedure can be done via your cervix or your abdomen, depending on which approach gives the doctor the best access to your placenta. It is generally performed between eleven and twelve weeks into your pregnancy, and the entire test is over within half an hour. We felt so blessed when we got the good news that Ashby's CVS did not detect any abnormalities.

CVS VERSUS AMNIOCENTESIS

There are several prenatal diagnostic tests. Two of the most common are the CVS and amniocentesis. You should talk to your doctor about the pros and cons of each. I chose to do a CVS because it was performed earlier in my pregnancy, and that way I could get results sooner.

How Ashby Got Her Name

Keith and I wanted to find out the sex of the baby ahead of time, and in our hearts, we both felt that we were having a girl. Keith already has two wonderful sons from his first marriage, and while he would have been happy either way, I knew there was a tiny part of him that wanted a girl.

Up until our second ultrasound, we had only ever discussed girl names. But after the technician told us she thought we were having a boy, we figured we'd better discuss some boy names, too. I pulled out a picture of my maternal grandfather whose first name was Ashby and said, "What about Ashby?" Keith loved it!

Six weeks later, I was exactly thirteen weeks pregnant. My doctor had the results of my CVS (chorionic villus sampling), which meant that he could tell us the sex of our baby. When we finally connected, he gave me the happy news that we were having a girl! Now we had to decide on a girl's name. Suddenly Keith said, "I don't care what you call her. But I'm calling her Ashby." "But that's a boy's name," I said. Then I looked up *Ashby,* and it turns out it's a dual-gender name that means "strength and courage." It was perfect.

What's in a Name?

Choosing the right name for your baby is a big deal. I bought several baby names books, and Keith and I spent hours going through them. Even though we ended up choosing a family name, I still recommend buying the books. They opened up the dialogue regarding what we were both looking for in a name. And it gave us the satisfaction that we had explored hundreds of names before we settled on *Ashby*.

Another way to come up with a meaningful name is to choose a place that holds significance for you and your mate. Keith and I tossed around Hawaiian names, because our first trip away together was to Hawaii. It was where we fell in love.

One more way to select a name is to find one that has a shared meaning for both you and your mate. For example: we added *Grace* as Ashby's middle name because not only was it the name of the church where my parents were married, Grace United Methodist Church in Union, South Carolina, but it was also the name of Keith's aunt.

And finally, once you settle on the name you intend to give your baby, I strongly recommend keeping it to yourself. We didn't, and had to hear comments such as, "Ashby? That will be confusing in school. It sounds like Ashley." But Ashley wasn't my grandfather's name, and I really didn't need to hear other peoples' opinions. So when it comes to your baby's name, do yourself a favor and take a vow of silence until the baby is born.

THE EARLY BIRD GETS THE WORM

Unfortunately, when my doctor called with my CVS test results, I missed the call because I was on the set. My fingers went to Speedy Gonzalez mode as I tried to call his office to catch him before he had left for the day, but alas, I missed him and got the "our office has closed for the day" message instead. I called back the next day, at exactly 9:01 A.M. sharp, one minute after the office had opened.

Listen, ladies. If you're waiting for results, it's best to call first thing in the morning. Doctors typically return their phone calls at the end of the day, which means if you miss their call, you might have to wait a whole other day (i.e., eternity) to get him back on the phone. So be sure to call your doctor first thing in the morning, when perhaps you can reach him before he sees his first patient. If he's already with a patient, then at least it puts you at the top of his callback list for that day. Just remember, the early bird gets the worm.

Fashionable First Trimester

Once you discover that you're pregnant, you don't have to run out and immediately buy a brand-new wardrobe. Your current clothes will pretty much last you through the first trimester, with perhaps a few modifications. These items and tips really worked for me. Hopefully they'll help you with your early pregnancy wardrobe, too.

* **Low-rise cords and jeans are perfect.** They can fit under the lower part of your belly.
* Pants with an elastic waist are great for the first trimester.
* **Drawstring pants are also very useful.** They can grow with you and can be let out as needed.
* You can hook a rubber band or hair band through the

buttonhole of your pants and use that to loop over the button. Couple that with a long, loose-fitting shirt and no one will notice that your pants are ever so slightly opened.

❋ **Get a belly band.** (It's like a tube top for the belly!) I can't thank my sister enough for this one! She mailed me a few of these as a pregnancy gift—and saved me a lot of money, because a belly band allows you to extend the life of your pre-pregnancy clothes. You put the band around your waistline and *over* jeans, skirts, and shorts that won't button because of your expanding belly. No one will have a clue that you're walking around with your pants undone because the belly band merely looks like a tank coming out from under your top.

❋ **Wear a long scarf.** Put it around your neck and let the two ends drape down to cleverly disguise your small baby bump. I used this trick while on-camera in New York, where I needed my scarf for warmth *and* secrecy. A large designer bag will do the trick as well, so this gives you a good excuse to buy one!

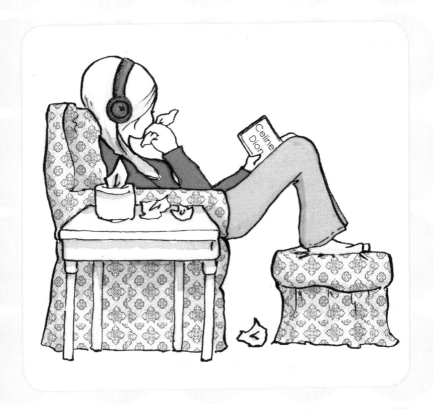

SECOND TRIMESTER

Now that you're in your second trimester (weeks fourteen through twenty-seven), you feel like you're out of the worry zone. You can officially start enjoying your pregnancy and sharing your news. And I was so excited, I shared my news everywhere, at all of the Hollywood events and to anyone who would listen—including Will Smith, who in his cute Will way said, "Gosh. I just thought you'd been drinking a little too much beer." (For the record, I don't even like beer.) And it's so nice after months to be able to tell people that, no, you're not simply gaining weight, you're growing a baby inside your belly!

At fourteen weeks, we planned to announce on air that I was pregnant. I was excited and nervous at the same time about sharing something so personal in such a public way. I knew that a few people I worked with had their suspicions, but overall I thought I had done a pretty good job of hiding my pregnancy. (Not the case.) After the announcement, the crew very sweetly presented me with an adorable outfit

45

they had bought for my baby (the cutest little boots and a onesie). Obviously, the cat had been out of the bag for quite a while. They had a present on standby!

Breaking It to Your Boss

A few weeks before I told the world, I sat down with my boss, Rob. I had been thinking for a while about how to tell him the news. Given the fact that I'm on-camera every day of the week, my pregnancy was something the producers needed to know about for a variety of reasons. As my pregnancy progressed, I wouldn't want to be working extremely long hours. I wouldn't want to be traveling like a madwoman. And of course, I would soon need a whole new wardrobe. My boss knew that Keith and I had been trying to conceive, but I wasn't sure how he would react now that I was officially pregnant. But when I told him, he was so happy for us (and I think maybe even happier for the show). I kid because Rob is my good friend, in addition to my boss, so he was truly ecstatic for us. But it was true that so many women in Hollywood were pregnant, and now, so was his host. It all was coming together like a well-produced segment. He joked that for the sake of the show I would allow a crew to film my delivery, right? Wrong!

I was happy and relieved by Rob's reaction, but I'd planned out what I wanted to cover during our conversation well in advance, to increase my chances that the news would go over well.

Here are some of the things I felt should be taken into consideration before sitting down with my employer. In case you're planning on having a similar talk with yours soon:

- ❋ Know ahead of time how much maternity leave you would like to take. I wanted to give my boss ample time to plan for my time away. If your work doesn't pay for your full maternity leave, consider using your paid vacation and sick days. (I used all of mine!)
- ❋ Understand your rights. I was so appreciative of Claudia, the head of our Legal Department, who told me about the Family and Medical Leave Act. Read it—it will help you to understand your rights as a new mom.
- ❋ Talk with your doctor. He may have an opinion as to how much time you should take off from work before and after giving birth.

EXERCISING WHILE PREGNANT

My whole life I've always been an avid runner, and during my pregnancy I asked my doctor about exercising. He shared with me his rule: for most women, if you were doing the exercise regularly *before* you got pregnant, you can continue to do it *while* pregnant (of course, we're not talking high-risk sports here). Unfortunately, several months before I got pregnant, I injured my back. So since I had not been running regularly before my pregnancy, I couldn't do it during my pregnancy. However, there are countless benefits to exercising while you're pregnant, and my doctor told me I could participate in these less intense forms of exercise:

* **Walking.** This works wonders for the cardiovascular system, is low impact, and is great for reducing swelling. Just watch the ground ahead of you as your belly grows bigger to avoid tripping on anything!
* **Swimming.** When you swim, you strengthen your muscles and increase your heart rate. Most fitness experts consider swimming the safest exercise for pregnant women.
* **Yoga.** This is a wonderful way to maintain flexibility with minimal impact to the joints, strengthen muscles, and relax.

A few other things I was told to remember: Be careful not to overheat; drink plenty of water; and be aware that as your pregnancy progresses, you're not as steady on your feet as you once were. And always consult a doctor before you embark on any fitness regimen.

Body Morphing

By the time I started my second trimester, my body was well into its baby prepping. During this stage I was amazed to see how much my body was changing on a day-to-day basis. Scratch that . . . on an *hour-to-hour* basis. I swear I looked more pregnant at the end of each day than at the beginning. It was wild.

I was thrilled, too, because so many of the issues that had dogged me in my first trimester had begun to settle down. For instance, my boobs didn't enter a room before I did. And I was no longer as sensitive to odors as I had been—Keith could once again wear cologne, and best of all, I could smell chicken again without having to run from the room. Sure, new things came up along the way (anxiety dreams, bouts of forgetfulness, and always feeling out of breath), but for the most part, I loved the second trimester, and there was a lot to love.

Second Trimester Plusses

My Skin

I swear it actually glowed. It was luminous and smooth. Now, you have to understand, every day I sit in a chair for over an hour while makeup is applied to my skin to create that *very same glow*! And at fifteen weeks pregnant, it was happening 100 percent naturally, all because of an increase in hormones due to my baby belly. I couldn't have been happier about it, especially since I'd read that an increase in hormones could sometimes cause the opposite reaction, aggravating skin and causing breakouts. Phew, I had dodged a bullet there. But then again, as my makeup artist would say, that's what makeup is for.

My Hair

I'd read, and friends had told me, that during pregnancy your hair becomes thicker, shinier, and more lustrous. But the truth is I didn't expect to see any significant change. My hair hasn't had a break from being styled in a long time—every single day, in order to get ready for the show, my hair is blow-dried within an inch of its life, which makes it dry and brittle. And yet, once I was pregnant, against all odds, my hair started to grow in beautifully. It was long, thick, and dare I say, lustrous.

COLOR ME MINE

When I got pregnant I wondered if I was going to have to go back to my natural hair color. What on earth would that look like? (Yes, I'm a bottle blonde.) I thought maybe hair dye (like skin products) could cross the skin barrier and be absorbed into the body, and with a baby growing in my belly, I didn't want to take any chances. So my hair colorist and I came up with a solution: We used foil strips to highlight, and he got as close as possible to my scalp without ever touching it. Even my colorist and I couldn't tell I wasn't having my base color done anymore.

Call Me Mama Bear

Around my fifth month I started to notice a real change in my personality. At some point your claws will come out, ladies. I've always been pretty easygoing and accommodating (it's the Southern girl in me). But all of that changed during my second trimester. For instance, if I wasn't given time to eat my lunch ... oh boy, look out! After all, I was eating for Ashby, too. And trust me when I say this, I am not a diva. Suddenly I was like this mama bear protecting her cub. There was a new sheriff in town. She was pregnant and she wasn't going to let anyone walk all over her. She would stop at nothing to protect her baby! I would hear myself speaking and I'd be like, *who is this?* Keith actually enjoyed watching me stick up for myself (and for Ashby, of course!).

Second Trimester Indignities

Forgetfulness

I'd heard that during pregnancy women can experience bouts of forgetfulness. But no one told me just how intense those bouts can be. I'd be in the middle of interviewing someone when all of a sudden I'd just plain forget what I was talking about. I'd drift into another world! All I can say is thank goodness the show wasn't live. Plus, basic everyday words started to elude me. I found myself asking questions like: "What's the name of that yellow fruit, shaped like a moon? You know, the one monkeys like to eat?" "Uh, do you mean a *banana*?" "Yes, that's it. A banana! Can I get one of those, please?" And at least once a week I'd "lose" my purse. I'd spend a half-hour walking around the office asking my co-workers, "Has anyone seen my purse? It's brown. It's leather. Kind of big?" Then someone would point to my shoulder, where my purse was hanging, assuming that this had to be some kind of joke—no one could be *that* forgetful.

However, I did remember to ask my doctor about my forgetfulness, and he said it happens to almost all his pregnant patients. Perhaps we're distracted or overwhelmed by thoughts of our new adventure. Regardless of the cause, there wasn't a darn thing I could do about it, aside from having the baby, and I wasn't ready to do that yet. So instead, per my doctor's advice, I just tried to relax and laugh about it. And I have to say, the unexpected bonus of forgetting basic everyday words was it forced me to think on my feet. I became the queen of synonyms, and I came up with some pretty hilarious ones during my pregnancy. When I couldn't remember the word for toothpaste, I described it to Keith as "creamy mouth medicine." Yes, I had temporarily forgotten the word, but he got the drift, and we never ran out of toothpaste.

Anxiety Dreams

At least once a week during the second trimester, I'd have a terrifying, panic-inducing nightmare. It would go something like this: I'm doing errands, proudly toting around my new little baby in her car seat. *She is so cute, so beautiful, so sweet, a bundle of perfection.* In my dream, I'm feeling like such a good mom when suddenly I look down and realize I don't have her anymore. I've left her somewhere. *But where? The makeup counter? The bank? The car?* And then I'd wake up panicky and anxious. Keith would have to reassure me. He'd say, "Honey, trust me. I promise you will not leave her anywhere." And of course, he was right. But I would still have those darn dreams throughout my second trimester. Meanwhile, my friend Stacie said she had wild and crazy sex dreams during her pregnancy (but *only* during her pregnancy). I really got the short end of the stick there.

Itchy Belly Syndrome

Okay, it's not really a syndrome. But wow, was my belly ever itchy. I had heard that women's stomachs can become itchy as the skin stretches across the abdomen, so I tried to head it off by moisturizing. I had my tubs of shea butter cream that I would religiously rub into my skin every night. But it didn't help. My doctor had warned me not to scratch excessively, because it could cause an abrasion, so Keith and I came up with the *towel technique.*

Here's how it works: Taking a towel, Keith would hold one corner in each hand, as if he were going to towel himself off. Then, standing behind me, he would flip it over my belly and, ever so gently, move the towel back and forth. Heaven, I tell you. Better than any cream. And better than doing it yourself! So my advice is: enlist a loved one and *gently* scratch that itch.

The Emotional Roller Coaster . . .

Well into my second trimester, I really didn't feel that pregnancy had changed my emotional state all that much. Sure, I would dissolve into a puddle of tears anytime Keith put the *Miracle* CD on. But how could I be held responsible for that? That whole CD is about motherhood, and I was about to become a mother!

I had been feeling pretty proud of myself: I wasn't moody or weepy, and overall, I'd been pretty even-keeled. I even once overheard my husband bragging to his friends how pregnancy hadn't changed his wife at all. "Look, at me," I thought. "I'm doing great. I'm totally in control." That is, until the great *paper towel incident*.

Keith and I were in the kitchen cleaning up after lunch, putting dishes in the sink and wiping down the counters. At one point, I dried my hands with a paper towel and left it on the counter. Keith turned to me and said, "Hey, babe, can you pick up that paper towel and toss it in the garbage?" And just like that, I started bawling. "How could you say that to me?" I sobbed. Keith's eyes went wide, like a deer caught in the headlights. "I didn't mean anything by that. Seriously, honey. I'll put the paper towel in the trash can for you." But it was too late. The tears were flowing—giant tears. "I can't believe you would criticize me like that!" Of course, no one was being criticized. I was just a pile of hormones. And the fact is, when it comes to pregnancy, you may think you're in control, but guess what? You're not in the driver's seat. Your emotions are at the wheel. So, buckle up!

Husbands Might Take a Ride, Too!

When I was twenty-seven weeks pregnant, Keith had to go to Vegas on a business trip, and he asked me to come along. His colleagues wanted to go to Celine Dion's show while we were out there, and they asked if I had an "in." I arranged for us all to go, and given my propensity for tears while listening to Celine, I gave my husband's co-workers a heads-up not to be alarmed if they saw me sobbing. (By now, I had started to carry a handkerchief with me.)

The concert started, and it was wonderful. Then Celine started into the song "If I Could." Are you familiar with it? Have you heard the lyrics? They're all about protecting your little one until he or she grows into adulthood. "If I could, I would try to shield your innocence from time . . . I've watched you grow, so I could let you go." *Let her go!* She hasn't even been born yet and already we're talking about her going off to college? As I was getting ready to pull out my tissue, I looked over at Keith so he could enjoy the entertainment. Could it be? Were those tears gathering in his eyes? Yes, they were. So, you see, those sentimental, runaway emotions aren't only for the ladies. No one is safe when that song is played.

Breathlessness

Why did I always feel out of breath, as if I'd just run up a flight of stairs? Perhaps I wouldn't have been so aware of it if I hadn't been on-camera, trying to interview Richard Gere in between huffs and puffs. Plus, during my pregnancy it was as if my voice had gone up an octave. I naturally speak in a deeper register to remove my Southern accent, but by my fifth month, I was breathing like a wild animal, y'all. I'm kidding, but still—no one mentioned that starting in my second month I might become a heavy breather. And it doesn't get better as your pregnancy progresses. Oh, no. Taking a deep breath becomes *more* difficult as your growing uterus starts to push up against your diaphragm, which in turn crowds your lungs (and makes doing a voiceover nearly impossible).

Say Good-bye to Your Lower Body

One day I woke up and I just couldn't see below my baby belly. My feet had disappeared. They were there the evening before, but the next day they weren't. Suddenly I had to strike these crazy poses in the shower, just to get water on my legs. Basically, my belly was acting as a giant rain shield for the lower portion of my body. And don't

Scaling the Second Trimester

By my fourteenth week, I was back on course and where I should be regarding weight gain. In the second trimester, an average pregnant woman will gain about one pound a week, and that's what was happening with me. Remember, eating for two (i.e., you and your unborn child) does not mean you need to eat twice as much. In fact, you should eat only approximately two hundred to three hundred more calories a day. And while most women have cravings—remember my thirst for milk and those circus animal crackers?—it's important to eat a well-rounded diet, which includes three servings of milk, yogurt, or cheese; three servings of fruits; four servings of vegetables; and nine servings of whole grains each day. But hey, even your doctor would agree, there's nothing wrong with the occasional donut for most pregnant women.

even get me started on shaving my legs. If I was wearing a skirt that day, I'd have to enlist my husband to do the honors. But on the plus side, it brought us even closer, and made for a great dinner party story!

Constipation

I was a big believer in not taking any medication during my pregnancy. So what was I to do about the constipation that pregnancy induces? (Yes, this lovely ailment comes as part of the pregnancy package. Lucky us.) First, I tried drinking prune juice. Yuck! Then I tried eating dried prunes. Yuck again! Finally, I had a great idea for how to get those needed prunes in my system without gagging: my mom's famous spice cake. Key ingredient: prunes. Key description: delicious.

My mother Betty's famous spice cake

2 cups self-rising flour

2 cups granulated sugar

1 teaspoon nutmeg

1 teaspoon cinnamon

1 cup vegetable oil (I use Wesson, which is what my mom used)

Five 2.5-ounce packages prunes (from supermarket's Baby Food section; look for "Stage 1." How appropriate!)

3 eggs (add them in slowly one by one as you're mixing)

½ cup chopped pecans (optional)

½ cup raisins (also optional . . . my mother-in-law Mama Z's suggestion)

First, preheat your oven to 350 degrees.

Using an electric mixer, beat together in a bowl the following ingredients: flour, sugar, nutmeg, cinnamon, oil, eggs, prunes, pecans, and raisins.

Transfer the mixture into two greased loaf pans (8 x 4 inches). Or, you can use one Bundt cake pan.

Finally, put in oven and bake for 50 minutes to 1 hour, depending on your oven.

Old Wives' Tales

When it comes to pregnancy, there are so many old wives' tales out there. "If you have heartburn when you're pregnant, you're going to have a hairy baby." That's so sweet. Just what every mother wants to hear. "If your linea nigra (the dark line that runs from your abdomen to your pubic bone) is straight, you're having a girl. If it's crooked, you're having a boy." And of course, "If you're carrying the baby in front, like a basketball, you're having a boy. If you're carrying low and your face looks fuller, it must be a girl"—because, as someone once told me, "Being pregnant with a girl sucks the pretty out of you." How nice. Thanks for sharing.

Once I was pregnant, I discovered that all bets were off. Everyone had an opinion and everyone was an expert. At *Access Hollywood,* my very creative executive producer, Rob, decided to make a little game of it. Once, when I was set to do the red carpet interviews at the Golden Globes, he decided that instead of doing the typical questions—tell me about what you're wearing, who do you think is going to win, etc.—he'd ask the celebrities to predict the sex of my baby. So, celebrities would stop to chat with us and would make their guesses. I was definitely carrying the baby right in front, like a basketball, so pretty much everyone thought I was having a boy. Will Smith: "Oh, it's definitely a boy! Clearly, a boy!" Eddie Murphy: "A boy. Yep. Absolutely. Tell him I said it when a boy comes out." The only person who had a differing opinion was Tony Shalhoub. He looked me up and down, then very thoughtfully made his prediction: "Nancy, you're having a girl. I just feel it." It was pretty impressive. Kudos to the casting director who cast him as *Detective* Monk!

It's Dizzying

Did you know that the pressure caused by your continuously expanding uterus can cause dizziness? It's true, so be careful when getting up. Another cause for dizziness in pregnant women is low blood sugar, so always carry a snack. (I toted a purse full of crackers and fruit. I thought of it as good practice for once Ashby was a toddler.)

Ring Around Your Collar

Don't be surprised if in your second trimester, your rings start to feel a little tight. It was during my sixth month that I noticed my fingers were starting to swell. If you have to take off your rings due to swelling, I recommend putting them on a chain and wearing them as a necklace, where they can stay close to your heart.

Gift Idea: The Ultra Frame

As your baby grows, the level of detail in your ultrasounds will increase. You'll be able to see little hands, feet, and your baby's face. I had the ultrasound that best showed Ashby's sweet face framed for my and Keith's parents, and I gave it to them as a Christmas gift with the words "Your Future Grandbaby" engraved on the frames. My mom placed theirs on the piano I played as a little girl. To this day, the framed ultrasound still sits there.

Showered with Gifts

If you haven't already registered at a store for baby items, the second trimester is probably the time to do it. The biggest recommendation I can give you is to get a friend who is a relatively new parent to help you. My friend Suzi Q was over at my house when I went online to register at a couple of stores. A mother of two young children, Suzi Q gave me great advice, such as:

✳ There's no need to register for cute little baby clothes, stuffed animals, and blankets. These are the most popular gifts, and you will receive plenty of them without adding even more to your collection by registering for them.

❊ Register for things people won't automatically think to give you, such as baby hangers (they aren't cheap), a second base for the baby's car seat (for Daddy's car), a diaper-disposal system, a babysitter chair (helps baby learn how to sit), baby carriers, handheld or plug-in nightlights, and baby socks (all your baby will wear on his or her feet the first six months).

❊ Consider registering for multiple strollers. They are a popular gift item and my friend Sonja told me I'd need various types of strollers—she was right. Depending on your lifestyle, you might consider registering for a travel stroller (it has a car seat that detaches from the base), a jogging stroller (it's easy to maneuver and it has big tires), or an umbrella stroller (great for when you're on-the-go, it's lightweight and folds up easily).

❊ If you can't resist and decide to go ahead and register for a few baby clothes, here are some suggestions:

- Register for older sizes, such as twelve months and older. The nursery closet will get filled with a ton of newborn-through-nine-month clothes, given as gifts. Babies grow so rapidly and are sometimes months ahead of the suggested age printed on the label.

- Register for soft clothes only. Some of the ornate outfits are darling, but your baby won't be comfortable in them.

- Consider clothes made from organic fibers, which are healthier for your baby.

Fashionable Second Trimester

If the first trimester is all about making your current clothes work for you, then the second trimester is about *finally* exploring the world of maternity clothes. Yes, that's right, you're now big enough to shop at maternity stores without feeling like an imposter. I couldn't wait to go to maternity stores to shop—there are so many, and the clothes are so chic now. Pregnancy has come a long way, baby! Here are some of my second-trimester shopping tips:

- **Buy bump-hugging clothes.** Maternity stores have incredibly gorgeous clothes these days that are designed to show off that bun in your oven. Now that you've told everybody, you want people to know you're pregnant, not bloated. So be loud and proud! I remember Halle Berry telling me she never felt sexier than when she was pregnant, and I felt exactly the same way.

- **Buy bottoms with an adjustable waist.** This was my favorite type of maternity clothes because they could grow with my changing shape. So clever! Look for maternity pants and skirts that have a hidden elastic band sewn into the waist, which can be cinched in or let out as needed by changing buttonholes.

❋ **Buy clothes in pregnancy-friendly fabrics.** Forget stiff or thick materials! This is especially important at the beginning of the second trimester, when your baby bump is not completely obvious but you want it to be. You don't want to look like you've eaten too many helpings, so stay away from materials such as cashmere, chenille, or wool, which add thickness and tend not to be flattering to your new curves. I recommend buying clothes in soft flowing fabrics made from jersey material.

❋ **Buy a pair of pregnancy Spanx!** Before I was pregnant I wore Spanx all the time. They help hold everything in place. So you can imagine when I got pregnant how thrilled I was to learn that they make Spanx for expectant moms, too. The pregnancy Spanx products hold everything in place, and feature a nonbinding waistband and stomach area, a soft, adjustable leg band, and added underbelly support. Hallelujah!

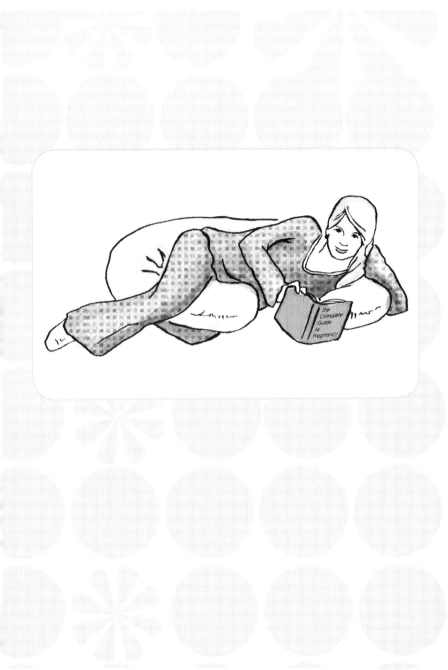

THIRD TRIMESTER

There are so many milestones in a pregnancy—from conception, to hearing the baby's heartbeat, to watching your belly take shape, to feeling the baby's first kicks. I was in awe of all of it. And as I entered my third trimester (which starts in the twenty-eighth week of pregnancy), I remember feeling a sense of accomplishment and pride. I was growing a beautiful, healthy baby in my belly. It was such a sweet time in life. And I'd never felt closer to Keith. One night, when we were in bed together watching TV, he looked over at me so sweetly and said, "Can you believe how soon we're going to have our little bambina right here with us?" He was so excited because he *loves* being a dad. That's one of the things that had made me fall in love with him—seeing him with his boys. Keith is the most incredible dad. And it's amazing to watch how much Carson and Tyler adore him. So I never had to wonder what kind of dad he would be to Ashby. I already knew: the best!

But I did have to wonder what kind of unexpected things would come up in the third trimester. And again, no one (not my friends, not the books, not even my *sister*!) had mentioned many of the things I would go through in my last trimester. To be fair, perhaps it's because leaky boobs and middle-of-the-night leg cramps aren't exactly life threatening to you or your baby, and therefore, not the first things on people's minds. But regardless, I would've liked a heads-up on some of these issues. For example, why didn't people tell me I would still need maxi pads when I was pregnant? I know what you're thinking, and you're right: you don't get your period when you're pregnant. But that, ladies, is not what you need the pads for. You need them for—and there's no other way to say it— pee! In other words, if you go to a funny movie and laugh really, really hard, you might wet your pants a little. And here's another tidbit about the third trimester: not only do your feet swell during pregnancy, but they *stay* swollen for quite a while after you give birth. Well, that was news to me. I knew I wouldn't be wearing my highest heels immediately after I had Ashby, but I liked to think that if I wanted to I could have. Not the case.

So here are the entertaining, often downright embarrassing, occasionally panic-inducing, but ultimately amazing things that happened to me during my last twelve weeks of pregnancy.

Sleeping on Your Side

There are many things a pregnant woman knows *not* to do. Don't drink alcohol. Don't eat unpasteurized cheese. Don't eat sushi. Stay out of hot tubs. Oh, and be sure to ease up on the skydiving. But in terms of how you sleep, none of my girlfriends ever said *one word* to me about what position I needed to sleep in: on my side, and specifically on my left side.

It wasn't until I was having a pregnancy massage that I learned how best to lie down when pregnant. I went to lie on my back when the massage therapist stopped me. No, no, I would need to lie on my *side*. "But wouldn't I be more comfortable if I were lying on my back?" I asked. And that's when she said, "Honey, when you're pregnant you're not supposed to lie on your back." What?! Wait, had I been sleeping on my back this whole time? Oh my gosh, my baby! The masseuse explained, "When you lie on your back, the pressure of your uterus can constrict the vena cava, cutting off oxygen to the baby. Now, relax and enjoy your massage." Relax? How on earth did she expect me to relax? All I could do was try to recall the number of times I'd woken up on my back. Finally, I came to the conclusion that I'm really a side sleeper anyway, and after the semi-relaxing massage, I went back home and did some research.

Turns out, the reason why the left side is preferred over the right is because it improves circulation to your heart and therefore allows for the best blood flow to the fetus, and your uterus and kidneys. So how do you ensure that both you and your baby sleep comfortably *and* correctly? Two words: maternity pillow!

To Snuggle or Snoogle?

The maternity pillow is a must. Run, don't walk to your computer and order one. At first I resisted—why did I need to purchase something when I could arrange all of my pillows around me like a nest? But inevitably I'd wake up, find the pillows scattered around the bed, and have to reassemble the puzzle. Finally I decided to throw money at the problem and buy a Snoogle (it looks like it sounds: a large pillow noodle). This pillow would quickly become my new best friend. It gave me a place to put my knees and it kept me comfortably on my left side. Think about it, your stomach is so big now that when you lie on your side, one knee is left to hover over the other. That's why the pillow is so great: It gives you a comfy place to rest your knee, plus it wraps around your back and prevents you from rolling over and . . . well, freaking out.

IMPORTANT SNOOGLE NOTE

The maternity pillow is huge and will take up the majority of the bed. By the end of my pregnancy, Keith was reduced to a tiny strip of the bed. But he was a good sport about it. It helps to remind your husband that it's only temporary—after the baby arrives, the foam snuggle husband you cheated with will be gone and you and your mate will have the rest of your lives to catch up on sleep. Yeah, right!

Foot Massages: Good in Theory, But Be Careful in Practice

The pregnancy massage therapist was a wealth of information. In addition to telling me about my sleep position, she told me to be careful when getting foot massages while pregnant because there are pressure points in the feet that are associated with the reproductive system, and overstimulation can induce labor. So make sure your masseuse is a *trained* pregnancy massage therapist, so your massage is relaxing *and* safe.

Leg Cramps

Some women have leg cramps during pregnancy. I had *lots* of them. One cause is the additional weight of pregnancy and the pressure from your growing belly on the nerves and blood vessels that go to your legs. I clearly remember the first one I had. I woke up in the middle of the night feeling as if my leg were in a bear trap. I punched Keith, and all I could say was, "Uh, oh, ow, oh, uh!" I couldn't get a single word out. All I could do was point to my leg and put his hand on my foot, motioning for him to bend it backward. It was like a painful game of charades. He finally got it. "Oh, you have a leg cramp! Yeah, those happen during pregnancy!" (Remember, he went through two pregnancies with his boys.) Wait a minute, now even my husband was on the "Why didn't you tell me that?" list.

But I forgave him because he got out of bed (and got *me* out of bed, which was not so easy at that point) to help me walk it off. Finally, I went back to sleep and woke up the next morning only to have the subject of leg cramps come up again with my mom-in-law (Mama Z, as I call her), who was visiting. I told her about my middle-of-the-night episode, and she said, "Oh, yes. I had cramps all the time when I was pregnant. I would wake up screaming!" Wait, even my mom-in-law participated in the "Don't ask, Don't tell" pregnancy policy? But once again, all was forgiven because, in the end, she came through with some great tips on how to help with leg cramps. And she should know. Keith is one of four boys, all one year apart. (Mama and Papa Z like to joke that they didn't have a TV in their bedroom.)

Mama Z's Recipe for Preventing Cramps

※ Stay hydrated. Drink *a lot* of water. Dehydration can cause the muscles to constrict, which in turn can trigger a cramp.

- Take a warm shower before bedtime. (This one really helped me.)
- Stretch your legs, especially your calves. No, you're not running a marathon, but if you don't stretch, in the morning, it'll feel like you did.
- Try eating a banana or a slice of cantaloupe or even a potato before bed. You might have mixed feelings about snacking moments before your head hits the pillow, but potassium is known to alleviate cramping, and those foods have loads of it.
- Sleep on your left side, which can help improve circulation for both you *and* your baby.

Mama Z's Recipe for Relieving Cramps

- Scream bloody murder. That way, you'll wake up your husband. Plus, it's good practice for when the baby screams in the middle of the night.
- Get your husband to massage your leg, no matter what time it is.
- Walk it off. For me, once I got a leg cramp, this was the *only* way I could get rid of it.

Scary Spots

I'll never forget the time my chest broke out in these little red dots. What the heck were they? I completely panicked. Did I have the chicken pox? They didn't itch, but whatever they were, they were all over my chest. I then spent an entire day, before I was able to get in to see my doctor, worrying about those spots. Well, thankfully after a visit with my doctor, I was told that what I was experiencing was absolutely nothing to be alarmed about. In fact, the red dots on my chest, also known as "spider angiomas," were due to high levels of estrogen associated with pregnancy. Ahh, those pesky hormones strike again.

My doctor explained to me that I had a 50 percent increase in blood volume due to my pregnancy, and therefore those red dots I was seeing were actually the ends of my blood vessels. He then assured me that while "spider angiomas" are not a very well documented aspect of pregnancy (I could've told you that), they were totally normal and would cause no harm to the baby. They would eventually go away . . . after I gave birth.

Hiccup, Hiccup, Hiccup, Hiccup, Hiccup, Hiccup . . .

Hiccup is a term used in TV production when you need to do something over. So it was quite ironic that we had to do a TV hiccup when I first felt my baby hiccup. I remember I was in the middle of an interview when I thought *I* had the hiccups! I just thought they felt lower than normal because I was pregnant. So I stopped the interview and said, "Wait, I have the hiccups." Johnny, the stage manager rushed out with water and then, as we all waited, I couldn't produce a single hiccup. *I* couldn't, because, as my doctor would inform me when I called him later, it was Ashby who had the hiccups!

Turns out, fetal hiccups are nothing to be alarmed about. In fact, my doctor said they're a good thing: it means that the baby has a functioning diaphragm. After Ashby's first in utero hiccup episode, I used to feel them multiple times a day. And I loved them! I felt like it was my baby's way of saying hi.

Springing a Leak

Who knew your breasts could leak even *before* you had the baby? Not I. Again, none of my friends decided to share this information, by the way. So, surprise, surprise, I had to find out the hard way.

The first time this happened to me, I was standing on the set, getting ready to read a story, when my cameraman, Kevin, panned his camera away. Then, Johnny quietly walked over to me. We've all worked together for years and those two are always protecting and looking out for me. So when Kevin quickly pans the camera away and Johnny walks over, that's my cue that something is out of place. You see, when we are taping the show, everybody on the entire NBC lot in Los Angeles *and* New York can watch. So, boy, do I depend on Kevin and Johnny. For instance, on many occasions, my Spanx will be popping out from under my skirt. Or my bra strap will be showing. Or, even worse, I might have more tan gel on one arm than the other. Horrid! But thanks to my guys onstage, those things usually remain between us. So when Kevin panned away this time, I checked for the usual culprits. But I couldn't find anything amiss.

That's when a team of stylists descended on me with hair dryers and Kleenex. Turns out, my boobs were leaking. Yes, horrifying, but true. Unbeknownst to me, dime-size wet spots had appeared on my blouse. Honestly, it was just like that scene in *Broadcast News* when Albert Brooks gets a case of flop sweat on-camera, and everyone is trying to dry him off before his next segment. In my case, it wasn't sweat. It was colostrum (or "pre-milk").

In the third trimester, be aware that your colostrum may come in. So you might want to switch to a thicker bra and buy yourself some nursing pads. They're like pillow-shaped maxi pads for your boobs. But when they're tucked inside a bra, no one will notice them. And Scout's honor, you'll never have to worry about wet spots again.

Did I Just Wet My Pants?

I started to notice during my last trimester that whenever I'd laugh, cough, or sneeze, I'd pee a little. It was totally embarrassing. I'm a grown woman who has been potty trained since she was two. And now suddenly I was wetting my pants? Well, it turns out, leaking urine— or "stress incontinence," as it is known—is a normal part of pregnancy. It's caused by the increased pressure of the uterus on the bladder. It doesn't seem fair, but it does make sense. So while it never completely went away during my last trimester, I did figure out a few ways to help reduce the number of wet spots.

❋ Try crossing your legs when you cough.
❋ Do your kegel exercises. Kegels are movements to help tone the muscles in the vaginal and perineal area. To do a "kegel," tighten the muscles around your vagina and anus. Hold this position for as long as you can (between eight to ten seconds) and then slowly release. These exercises will help to strengthen the pelvic muscles for birth and help minimize leakage.
❋ Limit the number of bladder-irritating beverages you consume, such as lemonade, coffee, and carbonated drinks.
❋ And, finally, stay on top of your bladder. For instance, if I knew I was going to interview Jim Carrey, I'd make sure to pop into the restroom first. That man is funny!

Do Your Doctor Diligence

At this point in your pregnancy you should think about lining up a pediatrician. It's best to do this *before* your baby is born—choosing a doctor is a hugely important decision, especially since you will visit the doctor's office at least six times for the first year of your baby's life.

That's why it's important to make a well-informed decision ahead of time. If you aren't sure where to begin your search, talk with your ob-gyn. Most obstetricians are more than willing to make a referral.

Another great resource is staff at the hospital where you intend to give birth. Otherwise, talk with your friends, neighbors, co-workers—really anyone you know who shares a similar outlook when it comes to children. I've gotten some of my best parental advice from friends.

Educate Yourself

You and your partner should definitely sign up for a birthing class (which are usually available at your hospital or birthing center), *especially* if this is your first child. Not only did it help prepare us for what to expect during labor and delivery, but it offered Keith concrete tips on how to assist me in a useful and effective way during labor. Keith is calm, cool, and collected anyway, but there were a few technical tips he added to his repertoire. I, of course, needed every morsel of information I could extract from the nurse teaching the class.

The nurse showed us a video of an actual birth and photos of newborns. And trust me, it wasn't the romantic comedy version. These images were graphic. There were shots of babies with cone-shaped heads, babies with birthmarks (also known as "stork's kisses"), and newborn boys with giant orange testicles. (Boy, was I relieved I was having a girl!) The nurse explained that if we were to see these things on our own baby, they were all *totally* normal. After all, as intensive and exhausting as giving birth is for the mom, it's also a tiring experience for the baby, who is being pushed and sometimes pulled through the narrow birth canal. We were also shown two additional videos, one of a woman who had been given an epidural before giving birth and one of a woman who chose to give birth naturally. Guess what? I liked the epidural version better.

The nurse also explained the correct way to push (think bowel movement—but we'll get into that later). Finally, she educated us on what would happen immediately after the birth, from cutting the umbilical cord to the baby being placed on the mother's chest.

Terrifying Terms

It was in the birthing class that I first heard the lovely terms "mucus plug" and "bloody show." The nurse rattled them off as if Keith and I used them as part of our daily lingo. So you don't have to look as shocked and terrified as we did, here are the definitions in brief: Your *mucus plug* is some sort of globular discharge that acts as a "cork" to your cervix. This may or may not become dislodged and may or may not be an indication of labor. Confusing, huh? Then there's your *bloody show*. No, it's not the midnight showing of *The Rocky Horror Picture Show*. Your bloody show is a pink-tinted discharge that indicates your cervix has begun to efface/dilate. If you experience a "show," you can expect to go into labor within twenty-four hours to a few days. So, there you have it.

Breast Feeding 101

If you intend to breastfeed (or, at the very least, give it the old college try), I strongly recommend sitting down with a lactation consultant, taking a class, or buying a book on breastfeeding *before* the baby arrives. Here's why: It's a lot harder than you think. Trust me. I speak from experience. I thought it was supposed to be all natural instinct taking over, with the baby suckling happily right out of the womb. Not quite! There's a whole technique to nursing, and you need to do it properly from the get-go or your nipples will get sore (*really* sore) quickly. So obviously there will be a learning curve, but waiting until the baby is born is too late. Educate yourself now.

Swell Advice

In the last eight weeks of my pregnancy, I started to notice that my shoes were feeling tight. Really tight. I wasn't wearing heels anymore because I didn't want to risk falling down. But even when I'd wear my "comfortable" shoes, it still didn't seem to do the trick. That's when I discovered that not only were my feet retaining fluid (known as "edema"), but they had also gone up half a size. Apparently, this can happen in the third trimester. I also made the upsetting discovery that it's not only your feet that can swell. One day, as I was getting ready for the show, my wardrobe stylists brought in these really sexy knee-high boots that went with a cute dress I was wearing. I tried to pull the zipper up, but after four inches, it stopped. I turned to them and said, "What are these, extra-skinny boots?" And that's when I got the *look* from Daniel and Nicole. The look that says, "It's not the boots that don't fit. It's you in the boots." And that's when I realized, it was my calves. So, yes. Sadly, your calves swell, too!

A Few Tips for Easing the Expansion

* Put your feet up as much as possible. It's no longer a recommendation, but a requirement. Doctor's orders. (You should have seen me in the makeup room with my feet propped up.)

* Again, sleep on that left side. It helps your kidneys efficiently eliminate waste products and fluids from your body. That, in return, reduces swelling.

* Avoid remaining in a standing position for long periods. This was a tough one for me, considering that we shoot the entire show standing up. I still remember the sweet crew members rushing in with a chair for me to sit on in between takes. (Thanks, fellas!)

- Exercise your feet often. Stretch them, spread your toes, and rotate your ankles as much as you can.
- When sitting, do not cross your legs as it can cause undue pressure on your feet and calves. (You should have seen me trying to look ladylike in my interviews without my legs crossed.)
- Try wearing maternity support hose, which can help reduce the swelling. Just be sure to put them on first thing in the morning, when you're your least puffiest.

Belly Souvenirs

Speaking of swelling, now would be a great time to make a souvenir of your ever-expanding belly. So get a belly-casting kit! In case you don't know, a belly cast is a plaster casting made of an expectant mother's pregnant belly. It's created by applying layers of wet plaster strips to the front of Mom's body. Once dry, the cast is removed, leaving a wonderful keepsake for you to share with your little one. It's a perfect way to celebrate the miracle of life. These kits are quite popular and easy to purchase online. Just make sure that the one you buy is made from 100 percent natural materials so that it's nontoxic and safe for Mom's skin. I always meant to do a belly cast, but I never did. I regret it to this day. You just never believe your belly can get as big as it does.

Another fun, and simple, belly souvenir is a piece of pretty yarn or ribbon the exact length of your belly's

Scaling the Third Trimester

By the time I neared the end of my third trimester, I felt huge. And it wasn't just my belly. Every part of me felt swollen. My breasts were enormous. My rings didn't fit. And my feet had gone up a size.

I had also gained thirty-one pounds, which was within the parameters of recommended weight gain, according to the experts. But still, I was curious, where did all of the weight go? I did some research, and found that the weight distribution for an average pregnant woman is:

7½ pounds (the baby's approximate weight at birth)

1½–2 pounds (the placenta)

4 pounds (increased fluid volume)

2 pounds (the uterus)

2 pounds (the breast tissue—mine felt more like 5 pounds for each breast)

4 pounds (increased blood volume)

7 pounds (maternal stores of fat, protein, and other nutrients)

2 pounds (amniotic fluid)

Grand total: 30 pounds

circumference at its roundest. My friend and co-worker Shaun Robinson gave me a wonderful shower at her house when I was nearing the end of my third trimester. She had so many fun games planned, and one was the "string game," where your friends guesstimate how big your belly is by cutting off pieces of yarn (without measuring it around you first, of course). That experience was quite humbling. Everyone guessed I was carrying sextuplets. Their yarn was all at least five to fifteen inches off! Except for one, my friend Lorrie, who won the prize. (Thanks, Lorrie, for not making me feel like a hippopotamus.) I kept Lorrie's piece of yarn, and it will be fun to pull it out someday and show Ashby how big my belly was when she was in it.

Feathering Your Nest

A few weeks before I had Ashby, I went on maternity leave from *Access Hollywood*. We had a few projects to take care of—namely, moving into a new house! Here's a big tip for you: Try to avoid moving into a new home in your final month of pregnancy. Talk about nesting! But all kidding aside, no matter where you are, if you're in an old house or new, you *will* get the urge to nest!

I was determined that my daughter's room would be ready by the time I gave birth. In fact, I went so far as to have some nursery furniture shipped to our new house while the current owners were still in it! (Thankfully, they were nice people and agreed to clear out that room first.)

I know some households have superstitions surrounding preparing for a baby before they come home from the hospital. But folks who don't share that belief are always anxious to start making arrangements for the nursery, and for good reason.

You Become a Turtle Toward the End

The closer you get to your due date, the more you start to sloooooowww down. You have less energy, less balance, less flexibility, and more weight. I went up and down the stairs at our new house so many times as I prepared the nursery that I actually fractured a bone in my foot. My body wasn't used to scaling heights with all that added pregnancy weight!

Paint Fumes

Paint the nursery as far in advance as possible. You want to make sure you give your baby's future room plenty of time to ventilate so the newborn baby is not exposed to harmful fumes. This applies to before the baby is born as well, because what you breathe, the baby receives. In other words, the safest route is to let someone else paint your nursery. Also, choose water-based, latex paints over oil-based ones. They contain fewer toxic chemicals— 50 percent fewer VOCs (volatile organic compounds).

Sorry, Baby, Your Crib's on Back Order

From the moment I knew I would be having a baby girl, I started envisioning what I wanted her nursery to look like. And I'm glad I did, because when I went to order Ashby's crib, changing table, glider, and ottoman, the salesperson told me they would take eight to ten weeks to arrive! I tried another company and was told the same thing. Then, when I ordered the material for the nursery curtains I found out that they were on back order as well. And my *second* choice for material had been discontinued. Was this a conspiracy? Not according to my designer, who said that material normally takes that long to come in. All of this would've sent me into an extreme panic had I not planned ahead. So, place your orders with enough time to allow for delays.

Making Sense of All the Material

I remember sitting on the floor of Ashby's future bedroom a few weeks before my due date surrounded by all of these pieces of cloth. One thing I discovered from my baby shower is that people *love* to give blankets—swaddlers, receiving blankets, burp cloths. Luckily, blankets make great gifts because you *will* wind up using them all once the baby arrives. But there I was, trying to make sense of all of these pieces of material, and I started to panic. *I don't know what to do with these things. Do I wrap the baby*

FULL *of* LIFE

88

in this? Or do I burp the baby with it? Is this something I'm supposed to wear when I'm nursing? Or is it meant to hang on the wall? I had no clue! I could feel my heart rate rising.

Thankfully, two friends of mine answered my panicked phone calls and came over for a blanket intervention. Together, we organized the nursery, tagged and labeled all of the clothes, and, along the way, they explained the differences between a receiving blanket and a swaddler. It goes something like this: A swaddler can be used as a receiving blanket. A receiving blanket can be used as a burp cloth or a changing pad. Even some burp cloths I was given were actually just decorated cloth diapers in disguise. It's kind of like Kevin Bacon's Six Degrees of Separation: they're all related somehow, and can be swapped in or out in a pinch. Phew!

Nursery Necessities

So, now you know not to buy blankets on your own; you will be given plenty. But here's a list of items that no one mentions you'll need and certainly no one will give you at your baby shower because they're not cute, tiny, soft, or cuddly, nor do they have lace trim. They're not fun to buy, and they definitely don't get "oohs" and "ahhs" at the shower. But once you have your baby, they're essential. And you want to stock up on these items *before* the baby arrives. Because the last thing you want to do after giving birth is run errands!

❄ **Gauze pads.** They're used to clean the baby's bottom the first two weeks. You can't use grocery store wipes at this point because a newborn's skin is too sensitive. I didn't know this until I was leaving the hospital. All I wanted to do was bring my baby home, but instead, we had to stop at the drugstore so Keith could run inside for gauze pads. So, take it from me. Stock up ahead of time.

❄ **Baby nail files.** Babies are born needing a manicure. Their fingernails grow in the womb, and by the time they're born, they need a serious trim. Otherwise, they'll scratch themselves. And trust me, it is too terrifying to use fingernail clippers on a newborn. Thank goodness I got a tip from a friend: buy some baby emory boards and have them on hand for when the baby is born. I didn't know they existed, but they do and they work like a charm!

❄ **Aquaphor.** Newborns tend to get eczema (a noncontagious rash that can appear on your baby's forehead, cheeks, and scalp). Ashby had a minor case of eczema. Her pediatrician recommended I get Aquaphor, and it helped to soothe her sensitive skin.

❄ **Thermometer head strip.** Now, no one wants to imagine their newborn getting a fever, but if we suspected Ashby might have one, we found this was the easiest way to check. All you have to do is place the

START DOING YOUR BABY'S LAUNDRY NOW

Don't forget to wash your baby's clothes *before* your little one is born. The reason: to remove any chemical traces, dyes, or little impurities that might irritate your baby's skin. And get this: you need to wash them in "baby detergent." When my housekeeper, Julie, mentioned this to me, I knew to listen. She's been with me for thirteen years and she always has solid advice. So, yes, even though I hadn't heard of it, detergent just for babies does exist. And I have to say, one sniff of it and I was sold. It was like the best perfume ever. *L'eau de baby.* Plus, it made everything feel so soft.

strip on the baby's forehead, and the thermometer gives you a reading by lighting up a color indicating normal to high temperatures.

※ **Moses basket.** This is where Ashby slept for the first six months of her life, even though she had the most beautiful crib! A nurse told me that newborns like small spaces, which makes sense. Think about it: they've been curled up in a ball in your belly for months. So lots of babies love to sleep in cozy Moses baskets. An added plus is that you can carry your baby from room to room in the basket without your little one ever waking up. I went through three of them!

※ **Bisphenol-A-free bottles.** You want to make sure that your bottles are polycarbonate free. Studies show that certain bottles, when heated, can release toxic chemicals, and the concern is that prolonged exposure to BPA in infants can cause developmental problems. Remember Abby, my pregnancy partner in crime? Well, she's the one who clued me in on getting BPA-free bottles. Again, it's great to compare notes with other moms.

What's Your Birth Plan?

I can't tell you how many times I was asked about my birth plan. Beyond giving birth to a healthy baby, I didn't have anything planned. Was I supposed to? Once again, I couldn't help but feel that I was missing something. So I called my doctor. Did I need to have a birth plan? And by the way, what the heck is a birth plan anyway? My doctor explained that it isn't mandatory to have a birth plan. But birth plans are an opportunity to think about some of your childbirthing decisions ahead of time, and to let the medical personnel know your preferences. He then asked me a bunch of questions. Did I want to give birth vaginally? Yes. Did I want to do natural childbirth? Absolutely not. I would be requiring an epidural. I don't like pain. Whom did I want to have in the room during the delivery? My husband. Could my doctor perform a c-section, if necessary? Of course. Whatever the doctor needed to do to ensure a safe delivery. I hung up the phone feeling much better. Yes, things might change along the way, but at least we now had a plan. So do you need a long written-out birth plan the way pregnancy books describe? If you'd like, but for us, our verbal birth plan was just fine.

Which Way?

Take it from me: take a tour of your hospital or birthing center *way* before your due date. We did it twice, and I am so glad we did. I will admit I have no sense of direction. With that disclaimer out of the way, I do believe a tour of the hospital to see the layout is a necessity. I gave birth to Ashby at Cedars Sinai in Los Angeles, which is a huge facility. (I even drew out a map of the hospital. Yes, I was a little paranoid, but what a comfort it was!) But whether you're delivering at a small or big hospital, it is important to know ahead of time which parking garage you're going to park in, which door you're going to enter through (and does this change if it's the middle of the night), what floor the maternity ward is on, and where you will check in. You already have enough to worry about; asking for directions shouldn't be on your list of labor to-dos.

Prepare Packets

Here's something else I prepared for ahead of time (I realize the following could be construed as somewhat anal-retentive, but I have to tell you, when my water broke and we were rushing to the hospital, it was nice not to be scrambling for important information): I made up information packets that I put in several key locations (i.e., my car, Keith's car, my suitcase, and another one in the kitchen, in case I went into labor when Keith wasn't there and someone else had to take me to the hospital). These packets contained vital information I would need for the big day:

- Copies of the pre-registration forms
- Copies of my health insurance information
- Directions to the hospital with alternate routes
- The map of the hospital (see "Which Way?")
- Important telephone numbers (i.e., my ob-gyn as well as those to notify when I went into labor—Keith's parents, my parents, my sister, Keith's brothers, my close friends, my boss

Fashionable Third Trimester

Well into my seventh month of pregnancy, I was set to host the Miss USA pageant in March 2007. Talk about needing some fashion tips! I knew I would be standing next to stick-thin beauty pageant contestants in swimsuits, and on top of that, this would be the first time in the history of Miss USA that a pregnant woman would host. Needless to say, I wanted to look my best. So I started to search for dresses. The one I liked the most was form-fitting and low-cut. Did I debate whether I should wear it? Yes. But I felt sexier than ever—I was finally at a place where, when you looked at me, you knew I was pregnant and I was loving it. In fact, one of the first things I said after opening the show was, "I'm pregnant and proud!" In addition to wearing what makes you feel good, here are a few tips for looking your best during your third trimester:

- ❄ **Black is best!** That was the color of the dress I wore to host Miss USA. It's classic, always in season, and very slimming, whether you're pregnant or not.
- ❄ *Do* **get a good pair of flats.** You will not want to wear heels at this point. You won't like the way they feel, and frankly, they're dangerous. They make you all off-kilter. If you go for sandals, buy strappy ones, which help disguise the swelling. I became obsessed with gladiator sandals in my last trimester.
- ❄ *Don't* **get a good pair of boots.** They probably won't fit. Remember when I told you that your calves swell in the third trimester? Don't waste your money.
- ❄ **Accessorize!** Put on a chunky necklace, some oversize earrings, and/or a scarf. This is a great technique to draw attention back to your face and away from your belly.

- **Leggings or stretch pants are perfect for pregnancy.** Couple those with a loose shirt or tunic, and you've got an adorable outfit. Plus, stretchy pants are something that can be worn from your second trimester through your third trimester (hopefully) and then be brought out again for those postpartum months.

- **Avoid cap sleeves.** In fact, avoid *anything* sleeveless at this point. Your arms are probably not your friends . . . especially at the *end* of the third trimester.

- **Pair solid fabrics with prints.** A head-to-toe printed dress can sometimes make you appear larger. I remember Gwen Stefani often paired a solid top with a printed skirt when she was pregnant, and it always looked flattering and hip.

It's almost time!

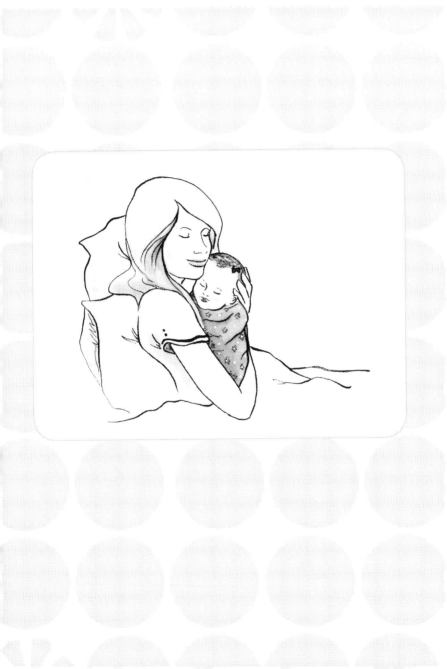

LABOR, DELIVERY, AND THE HOSPITAL STAY

By the night of June 10, 2007, my due date had come and gone. Well, almost. Around nine o'clock, I was sitting in the living room with Keith, my two stepsons, and my mom and dad, who had flown in from South Carolina the week before. We all started speculating about how much longer it would be until the baby arrived. Obviously, I knew I was close. In fact, my belly had continuously been dropping for the past two weeks, like the crystal ball in Times Square on New Year's Eve. Was tomorrow going to be the big day? Or the next day? Everyone started to place their bets. Tyler was certain I was going to go into labor that night—at 3:00 A.M., to be exact. Since my dad's birthday was the next day, on the eleventh, Dad was hoping that Ashby would be born then. I had to agree that it would be so darn cute to have Ashby's birthday on the same day as my dad's, and hoped it would turn out that way.

As the conversation began to wind down, I turned to my mom, who was sitting next to me holding my hand. It's hard to explain, but my body was definitely feeling *really* different at that moment. There were some physical components to the feeling. I was ever so slightly crampy, like when your period starts. But mostly I was feeling different *emotionally*. A calm, new sense of purpose had come over me. I squeezed my mom's hand tightly and said, "I just feel in my heart that tonight is the night." Call it soon-to-be-mother's intuition, but I had an instinctive feeling that it was time. My mom then told me that she had that same feeling.

Well, if my mom was saying that she thought I was going to have the baby that night, then I was having the baby that night! You see, my mom and I have always had a special connection. We used to talk every day on the phone, even though she was in South Carolina, and many times when I called, the phone wouldn't even *ring* on her end because she'd already picked it up to call me.

MOTHERS AND DAUGHTERS

I firmly believe that there's an almost telepathic connection between mothers and daughters that starts before birth and lasts throughout a lifetime. That's why I think I knew that Ashby would be born the night she was. And my mom always had an uncanny sense when it came to me. In fact, she somehow knew the day I was going to meet Keith. I had been having a bad week, and my mom and dad were going to come for a visit until, uncharacteristically, my mom called me as I was heading to the airport to go on a quick business trip and said, "I don't think your father and I should come out this time because I feel like you are going to meet someone you're supposed to meet. And if we're there, you won't go out with them." A mere ten minutes later, I met Keith in the security line at the airport! Sometimes her feelings were so dead-on it was spooky. In other words, if she thought something was going to happen, I knew I'd better sit up and listen.

So after my talk with my mom, I went upstairs to prepare. I took a shower, made sure my information packets were ready, and zipped up my suitcase and put it near the front door. Tonight was the night!

Hospital Checklist

Packing for the hospital is one of those things that's actually trickier than it sounds. You don't want to overpack (you're there for only three to four days, depending on the type of birth you have), and yet you want to make sure you have all of your creature comforts. Plus, your post-baby needs are different from your pre-baby needs. Then, factor in the fatigue and forgetfulness that haunt all pregnant women. This is why I recommend compiling a list. And just like Santa, check it twice.

Of course, Keith kept assuring me that he could always drive back to the house and get whatever I needed, but I knew I wouldn't want him to leave the baby and me. So I made sure my list was thorough. Here's what was on it:

- ❋ **Pre-registration forms.** Remember those information packets I told you about? Each packet included my pre-registration forms, my insurance information, my health history, and doctor's contact information. Now is your time to pull out those packets and use 'em. I put one in the outside pocket of my suitcase. When I got to the hospital, I handed the packet to the maternity check-in person. It contained everything they needed.

- ❋ **Nightgowns and pajama bottoms.** I recommend treating yourself to several new comfortable, yet pretty nightgowns—nothing you'd catch your granny wearing—*with easy access for nursing.* If you choose to breastfeed (which I highly recommend as I found it to be such a bonding experience), look for gowns that have buttons down the front. I recommend bringing three to four nightgowns to the hospital and having two to three in your closet at home. The last thing you want to do your first week home is laundry. Also, pajama bottoms are great to wear under your nightgown, both to stay warm and to help keep your maxi pad in place. Be sure to bring four to five pairs to the hospital. The pajama bottoms will also provide an additional layer for leakage, so you want to have more than one pair per day—because, though I hate to say it, there will be leakage after you've given birth.

❋ **Breastfeeding items.** Speaking of leakage, you will also have some from your boobs. So, you need to pack nursing pads (see pages 77–78 for more info on these). Also, be sure to take lanolin ointment, to prevent your nipples from cracking, and soothing breast gel packs in case your nipples get sore. (Mine were sore from the beginning.)

❋ **Full-coverage underwear.** Trust me when I say this, you'll want to pack underwear with full coverage. And lots of it. This is no time for thongs, ladies. You will not be thinking about panty lines post-labor. You'll want underwear that is both comfortable and that can accommodate a maxi pad—a *big* pad (like a king-size pillow). Also, make sure the elastic isn't too tight. Depending on what kind of birth you've just had, you might not want anything snug around your pelvic area.

❋ **A pillow (and pillow case) from home.** Hospital pillows can be lumpy and thin, so I recommend bringing a plump one of your own. Plus, it's comforting to have something that smells like home. But don't forget to take it with you when you check out!

❋ **An outfit to wear home from the hospital.** I brought a nice baby pink Juicy Couture sweatsuit to wear home. (I even coordinated my outfit with Ashby's, which was a precious layette set, white with pink trim. But we'll get to that later!) Now remember—and this is important—you will look like you're about five to seven months pregnant *after* you've had your baby. So make sure that the clothes you've picked out to wear home are items you were able to wear during your second trimester. I remember my dad teasing me when I got home from the hospital. "Are you sure you weren't supposed to have had twins? Because I think you still have another baby in there." Thanks, Dad. I had *no* idea I would be that big when I left. So brace yourself, and leave your skinny jeans at home.

❋ **Makeup.** When I packed my makeup bag I remember thinking, *this is going to be the last thing I'm going to feel like putting on.* But my makeup artist, Karen, recommended I bring some. And she had a great reason: You're going to want to take pictures with your new baby. Lots and lots of pictures. These are photos you'll keep forever. They might even make it into a prominently displayed frame. So you don't want to look tired. I mean, of course, you are going to be exhausted. But you don't have to look it. And this is where a dab of blush, a swish of lip gloss, and some mascara come in. You might also consider bringing a handheld mirror so you can actually see where you're applying the makeup, because you probably won't feel like standing up and heading to the bathroom. I didn't. And if you've had a c-section, you might not even be allowed to get out of bed. But I swear once you have a little bit of color on your face, it'll make you feel so much better.

❋ **Batteries, memory cards, extra videotape, and chargers.** Okay, so you've packed your camera, video camera, and cell phone. But have you packed your memory cards, extra videotape, and chargers? This is the critical stuff! From the moment Ashby was born, Keith and I were capturing every cry, coo, stretch, and eye flutter with our camera, video camera, and BlackBerry. And as soon as Keith was done taking pictures, he was downloading them and sending them off to friends. (Which reminds me, bring your laptop!) If we had forgotten our batteries, chargers, memory cards, or extra videotape the entire operation would have come to a screeching halt. So after you've packed all of your gadgets, go back and make sure you've packed all of the things that keep those gadgets going!

❋ **Car seat (with infant-head-support insert).** In order to take the baby home from the hospital, you need to have a rear-facing car seat installed. It's the law. So make sure you have it put in before your due date. And here's a handy tip: If you're having trouble figuring out the correct way to install the car seat (or you're not quite sure that this is your partner's area of expertise), stop by your local police precinct. The cops are trained in installing car seats, and are more than happy to do it. Who knew the boys in blue could do that?

Also, remember: The car seat should be installed in the middle of the backseat. Why the middle? It would be the safest place for the baby if you were to have an accident. (But I promise you, your ride home from the hospital will be the *slowest* and the safest you and your mate have ever driven with your new bundle in the back. I swear it took us an hour to travel seventeen miles!) And one more thing: If your car seat doesn't come with one, you need to make sure you've bought an infant-head-support insert. This provides your baby with extra head, back, and neck support. So buy it and give yourself peace of mind.

CAR SEAT TUTORIAL

Once your car seat is installed, take a moment to learn how to adjust the straps. Most car seats have the straps factory adjusted to their tightest level, and you'd have trouble squeezing a teddy bear into one, let alone a baby. So familiarize yourself with how to loosen the straps ahead of time, so when you're finally ready to bring the baby home from the hospital (which is stressful enough as it is), you won't be battling with the car seat straps on top of everything else.

Popping

I was ready. Everything was packed and ready to go. And at 3:00 A.M. on the nose (good guess, Tyler!) I was lying in bed, trying to get comfortable when, all of a sudden, I felt a pop. If you're curious what it feels like when your water breaks, to me, it felt like a bubble gum bubble had just burst inside of me. It was a small, painless sensation, but definitely a pop. I tapped Keith. "Babe, I think my water just broke." He opened his eyes and shook his head. "No, it didn't. Trust me. Just try and get some rest." Remember, Keith had already been through this twice before with the boys, and he felt he knew the drill. But I knew something was going on. "No, seriously, I'm sure of it. My water just broke." By now I was up and out of bed. Keith was following a few steps behind, still skeptical. "Sweetie, if your water broke, we would see something." And as if on cue, water started trickling down my leg. Aha! "See that, I told you. My water *did* break." Then all of a sudden, it hit me. *Holy moly, my water broke! I'm having the baby! We've got to go!* I didn't want to be one of those women who accidentally gave birth in the car on the way to the hospital. I had a plan and it involved my doctor, the hospital, and an epidural!

We called my doctor's office and were told to head to the hospital. Everyone—Keith, my doctor, the nurses—was so calm, which was reassuring. We woke my parents to tell them what was going on, then grabbed my suitcase, loaded it in the car, and headed to the hospital. It was showtime!

Go with the Flow

I was surprised to learn that only one in ten women experiences her water breaking *before* labor begins. And some women never experience it at all, ending with the doctor having to rupture the amniotic sac.

While my water did in fact break, it was not at all the way I'd imagined it. I thought there would be this huge rush of water, like the Hoover Dam had broken. In fact, I was so paranoid about the possibility of my water breaking in public that I had actually stopped going to restaurants and movies as my due date approached. Of course, when my water eventually did break, it was nothing like that. It wasn't an epic release of water; it was more of a trickle, thicker in consistency than water, with some red streaks in it that indicated it was amniotic fluid. I knew to look for the streaks because, prior to my water breaking, I had asked my doctor how I would know for sure if it happened. He told me that aside from the color, amniotic fluid smells kind of sweet (unlike urine, which has more of an ammonia-like odor), and that it will *continue* to leak. When your water breaks, you should call your doctor, and be sure to keep the area clean to avoid infection. Grab a maxi pad to absorb the flow, and then get in your car and head for the hospital.

Labor of Love

By the time Keith and I arrived at Cedars Sinai Hospital, it was four thirty in the morning. Shortly after we arrived, the nurse hooked me up to a monitor, turned to me, and said, "Did you know you're already having major contractions?" I couldn't believe it. "I am?" The nurse nodded. They didn't feel like major contractions. Weren't contractions supposed to be painful? Wasn't I supposed to be screaming at the top of my lungs and gripping my husband's arm? I mean I was feeling *something*. But in my case, it was more like a heavy menstrual cramp than searing pain. The nurse then gave me an exam. My cervix had begun to dilate (open) and efface (thin out). Things were progressing nicely. Everyone was so calm and civilized (including me!). This was nothing like an episode of *ER*.

Time and Time Again

After my exam was over, another nurse led us to our "labor room," and she informed me that my doctor would be in to see me at 7:00 A.M. *What?!* I panicked. *But that's two hours from now!* Yes, that's right: In most traditional, non-emergency deliveries, you will not see your doctor until you're in "active" labor (i.e., your cervix has dilated to seven centimeters). Oh, and FYI: You don't give birth until you've dilated to ten centimeters. The nurse calmed me down and told me we still had, "Plenty of time." *Plenty*

of time would become a phrase that was uttered to us over and over again.

I had had this image that we would be rushing—that my contractions would be excruciating from the get-go, and within a matter of hours, I would be delivering the baby. No, no, and no! It was totally the opposite. I wasn't in major pain. Everyone was totally calm. I walked around the floor for a while. I even had a Popsicle. We did, in fact, have *plenty of time.*

Pito-what?

A few hours into my labor my doctor set up an IV drip to administer Pitocin, which is a synthetic hormone used to induce or hasten labor. Since I was already in labor, it was being used to gently but effectively speed things along. Most doctors want you to deliver the baby within twelve to twenty-four hours after your water has broken, because of the risk of infection for both you and your baby. A rupture in the amniotic membrane opens the way for germs. Hence, the need for Pitocin.

What Contractions Feel Like

I had never been in a room when someone gave birth, so my expectations about labor and contractions were based on movies and TV shows. I thought I would be screaming bloody murder when I had a contraction. The

Pitocin had sped up the contractions, and they definitely

hurt, no question about that. But they weren't *ridiculously* horrible, at least not for me. I would feel them coming on and tell Keith I needed his hand. I'd squeeze it while concentrating on something pleasant, and then, in a few seconds, the pain would be gone. To me, contractions felt as if someone were screwing something tight around my abdomen, then tighter, then tighter, then even tighter, and then . . . released. They were certainly manageable, and I tell you this because the mind can make things better or worse, depending on your outlook.

With my contractions growing stronger, my doctor, like a knight in shining armor, finally arrived. He reassured me I was doing great, and things were progressing nicely. He then told me I could've gotten my epidural by now. I explained that I had held off because I knew that once I got the epidural I would have to stay in bed (as the epidural requires frequent blood-pressure monitoring, and continuous fetal monitoring), and I had wanted to walk around. He said, "Well, we're close. You're going to deliver at around twelve thirty. So if you want one, you can go ahead and get it." Yeah, I'll take that epidural. And let me tell you . . .

I Love Epidurals

I'm not someone who likes pain. But it wasn't until I was close to delivering (or, to be exact, at Phase Three, wherein the woman's cervix dilates to ten centimeters)

that I could understand why someone *might* want to screammmmm! That's when I knew, my time had come. Relief was on the way.

Once the epidural had been administered (by the way, it's given to you through a needle inserted into your spine), I literally felt no pain. Nothing. It was kind of surreal—Keith and I would watch the monitor in order to know when I was having a contraction. After the epidural, that was the only way to know when one was coming! It was wild, and all I can say is, thank goodness for epidurals.

Wait . . . This Is It?

I had this idea of what my birth would look like, and it involved multiple doctors bustling around me, with nurses everywhere, but our experience couldn't have been further from that. Our doctor sat on the edge of the bed and talked with us as if we were friends hanging out at a barbecue. Then he leaned in and said, "Okay, Nancy, it's time to start pushing." "Push . . . as in the baby?" I asked. He nodded. I couldn't wrap my mind around what he was saying. "Wait, this is it?" I asked. He nodded again. Then, my doctor, who had been sitting with us just wearing his shirt and tie, put on his white coat and rubber gloves, and called over the nurse. What about the *nurses plural? Aren't there supposed to be more than just two of you in here with me?* Well, if you have a c-section, there's *way* more than two, but if you give birth vaginally, your entourage is pretty small. With the help of my little team, I was coached to push, and then after about five contractions and pushes, I heard Keith yell, "I see her head!"

LIGHTENING UP

At my last visit with my doctor before the birth, which took place early in the week of Ashby's due date, he told me that Ashby's head had settled nicely into the birth canal. This is called "lightening" or "dropping." He also referred to it as Ashby being "engaged." (*Engaged?!* Oh, Daddy Keith was not gonna like this.) He told me that Ashby would most likely maintain this position until birth, and the fact that her head was down and already engaged was a good thing, and would most likely make my delivery easier.

You Should Know

After about twenty-five minutes of pushing, my doctor said, "With a couple more good pushes, Nancy, I think you'll finally be able to meet your baby girl." I couldn't believe it. It was all so much simpler than I had pictured. My husband always says I shouldn't say that, because other women who have had a more difficult labor might not like it. But I think the *positive* stories should be out there, too! So here, I'll say it: my labor and delivery were not all that

LABOR, DELIVERY, AND THE HOSPITAL STAY

difficult. Uncomfortable, yes (only before the epidural). But difficult, no. And I hope yours is the same!

A FEW WORDS ON PUSHING

The nurse who conducted our birth class gave me a fabulous tip about pushing. She told me that one of the biggest mistakes women make during their delivery is that they push with their faces—teeth clenched, eyes bugged out, screaming at the top of their lungs. But that's totally the wrong way. It does you no good, and by pushing that way, you might break blood vessels in your eyes and face and give yourself a monster headache and a swollen face. Instead, you want to push as if you're having a bowel movement. Yes, it's true!

It's Nice to Meet You

After a few more pushes—about thirty minutes of pushing, total—I heard Keith say, "Oh my gosh! Oh my gosh! Here she comes, babe! Push hard! Push hard!" And then the moment I had waited for for so long had finally arrived. I heard my daughter's first cry. I cannot begin to describe the feeling of what it's like when you hear your baby for the first time. They're no longer communicating with you from inside your body. They're out and letting the whole world know it. I was so overwhelmed with emotion and love.

And Then She Looked in My Eyes

It's hard even to put into words what happened next. I can tell you *technically* what I witnessed: The nurse suctioned Ashby's nose and mouth in order to remove excess liquids and to clear her breathing passage, and all the while she was still letting out that newborn cry. (*That* part was just like I'd seen in the movies.) But this next part you'll just have to experience yourself in order to understand the elation it brings. The nurse put Ashby on my chest and immediately my little girl became completely quiet and looked me directly in the eyes, almost as if to say, "Hi, Mama. I know it's you and I love you." No introductions necessary. There it was: that instinctive mother-daughter bond was happening. I could feel my heart grow!

DOCTOR'S ORDERS: SNUGGLE

After a vaginal birth, babies are often placed immediately on the mother's abdomen or chest. This helps to begin the bonding process and also helps keep your baby warm.

We Scored!

After we bonded for a few minutes, Ashby's umbilical cord was clamped in two places (Keith did the honors and cut the cord). Then, the hospital put on her ID bracelet and checked to make sure it matched mine. (I was happy to see them do that! This baby was *mine*.) Next, she was cleaned up, measured, and weighed. Ashby weighed seven pounds, nine ounces, and was twenty-two inches long. The doctors administered the Apgar test. In case you're unfamiliar, the Apgar measures "appearance," "pulse," "grimace," "activity," and "respiration," and is a quick test given one minute after the baby's birth and then again, five minutes later. Ashby got a good score. We were very proud.

A CUTE GAME FOR THE MEN IN YOUR LIFE

Here's something the fellas in your life can do that'll give them yet another reason to be excited about the baby's arrival. (Keith, his three brothers, and his father invented this game over Thanksgiving.) Guess what the length and weight of the baby will be at birth. Each guy puts his guess in an envelope and seals it. Keith, his brothers, and his dad talked and debated about the bet from Thanksgiving all the way through June, constantly evaluating *my* size to see if that would clue them in as to who would win. (Just what a woman wants: a bunch of men talking about her weight and stomach size!) Guess who won? Keith! And not only

Afterbirth

Did you know that after your baby comes out, you still have to give birth to something else? That's right. The final stage of childbirth involves the delivery of the placenta, or afterbirth. It happens right after the baby is born and takes only five to ten minutes. I didn't even realize it was happening! I was just holding Ashby in my arms, counting her cute little fingers and toes, when my doctor said, "Great. Your placenta is out." I didn't even know he had been pushing on my abdomen, helping it along. I couldn't have cared less at that moment, because I had my prize, my sweet baby. And nothing could distract me from her.

The Scoop

When I was talking about labor and delivery with my girlfriends, my friend Leah, who has absolutely no filter when it comes to telling it like it is, added, "Oh yeah, and don't be surprised if you actually poop on the table." Excuse me? I remember lying on the table getting ready to have Ashby, when I worked up the nerve to ask if this was true. "Could this happen?" I asked the nurse. "And if it did, how do you keep it sanitary?" The nurse replied, "Oh, yes, honey. It happens all the time. Remember, you're supposed to push as if you're having a bowel movement. But, no worries. We're set up for that. We have a pad and we just zip it off and zip a clean one back on. And you'll never even know what happened." Well, that was a relief, I guess. Of course, after Ashby was born I had to ask. "So . . . did I?" The nurse told me that I had not, but I sure pushed as if I were going to!

Wait a Second . . . Where Did That Hair Come From?

When Ashby first came out and the doctor held her up I was immediately, completely in love with her, and I thought she was the most beautiful baby I had ever seen. But wait a minute—she has jet-black hair! Where on earth had that come from? Keith has light hair, and I'm blonde. I turned to Keith and jokingly said, "I swear I didn't fool around with the milkman, babe." I had pictured in my mind a thousand times over holding my brand-new *blond* baby. I didn't care either way—the only thing that mattered, of course, was that she was healthy, which she was. But it was such a shock! I'd always assumed her hair would be blond. And then it dawned on me: I *do* get my hair highlighted . . .

Within a couple of months, Ashby's hair lightened up. And if you think about it, it makes sense that her hair was dark when she was born—a baby's hair hasn't seen a ray of sunlight because he or she has been inside of you. But what a shocker for me!

After the Baby Is Born

We "roomed in" with Ashby. In fact, the hospital told me that if we so chose, she could always be with one of us. And she was, which was a relief, especially for someone who has watched one too many movies of the week—I didn't have to worry about a possible mix-up of babies or about her getting taken from the hospital. (Yes, I'm a little paranoid.) Most hospitals allow babies to "room in" with their parents, especially if there are no complications. So if you want that option as well, ask your hospital.

Ashby was with me throughout the entire hospital stay, except for one hour, when she had to get her newborn screening tests. But Daddy Keith was by her side during those. By the way, Keith said those tests are a little traumatic for dads, because the baby's finger is pricked and gets squeezed and squeezed and squeezed so the doctor can get several blood samples. Now, I know those tests are necessary to ensure the health of the baby, but I certainly was glad when she came back. Having Ashby in the room with us was wonderful—we could bond, and I was able to nurse her on demand. Speaking of nursing . . .

Breastfeeding Is Tougher Than You Think

The nurses suggested that Ashby and I get started breastfeeding right away—within an hour after she was born. *Great,* I thought, assuming breastfeeding was going to be easy. I had no clue that there was a whole technique behind it. It's called "latching," as in latching the baby onto your breast. The baby will naturally open her mouth when you brush her lips across your nipple. When her mouth is open and tongue down, you quickly have to bring your baby to your breast (not your breast to your baby), and the mouth has to be open wide enough to cover your areola, not just your nipple. (If you let your baby suck only your nipple, it will get really sore.)

I didn't latch properly at first because I waited for the lactation consultant to come on day two of my stay at the hospital, and by the time she arrived, my nipples were on fire. And when I say on fire, I mean four-alarm! Thankfully, she taught me the proper way to both latch on and latch off. *Wait, there's a technique to latching off, too?* Yes, if you pull the baby off abruptly, it can cause injury to your nipple. Instead, you break the suction by putting your pinky into the corner of your baby's mouth, to admit some air.

The lactation consultant also taught me the various nursing positions. There's the cradle hold, the crossover hold, the side-lying hold, the tailor hold—what are these, football plays—and, yes, the football hold. Bottom line: You can see why it would be extremely helpful to get breastfeeding advice *ahead* of time. This was a lot of information to take in. I wish I had known a little more before game day, and I highly recommend speaking to a lactation consultant *before* you give birth.

Have Patience

So what happens if you don't latch properly at first and your nipples are on fire like mine were? Do you have to live with that excruciating pain for the duration of your nursing? (I swear it was worse than contractions for me.) The answer is *no*! My advice is very simple: Have patience and don't give up, because there is light at the end of the tunnel. I had a friend tell me, "Nancy, if you can hang on and continue to nurse for three weeks, I promise you your nipples will toughen up and the pain will subside." And she was right.

Somewhere between two and three weeks, the pain completely disappeared and I was so glad I persevered for Ashby, because breastfeeding is so healthy for her. Note: During that waiting period, pull out those soothing cool breast gel packs for your nipples I told you about on page 105. They were heaven-sent!

SMALL APPETITES

Did you know that when a baby is born her stomach is the size of a marble? Meaning, newborn babies don't need as much food as you think. They typically can get all their necessary initial nourishment from your colostrum (also known as "pre-milk"), which your body produces until your milk comes in (usually on the third or fourth day after delivery, although mine came in on the second day. Everyone's different).

The Doctor Is In

Within twenty-four hours of her birth your baby will be seen by a pediatrician. This will be either the doctor you've chosen or the on-call doctor at the hospital. During the visit, the doctor will make sure your little one has no congenital abnormalities, is feeding adequately, and is bonding with you (the mom). In addition, your baby will be given a head-to-toe physical exam. I suggest having a list of questions written out ahead of time that you can ask during this visit. As you can imagine, I had quite a long list. I wanted to know how often I needed to breastfeed, how I would bathe her, how to care for her umbilical cord, and even how often she was supposed to poop and pee. (Remember, you'll be keeping track of this!) The doctor will greatly appreciate your questions, and may have additional things to tell you.

You Are the Sunshine of My Life

When the pediatrician told us that Ashby had a little bit of jaundice, I couldn't believe what I was hearing. The doctor, who had already rightly me pegged as a worrywart, quickly assured us that it was *nothing* to worry about. In fact, 50 to 60 percent of babies have a yellowish tint to their skin in the first one to two weeks of life. I wish I had known beforehand that this was so common, because it really scared me when the doctor told us.

Jaundice is brought on by an excess of bilirubin, a pigment in the blood that causes the skin to look yellow. But Ashby didn't look particularly yellow to us. The pediatrician explained that most babies have some sort of jaundice, even if it isn't visible to the naked (or untrained) eye, and that jaundice is a temporary condition. Ashby's would most likely go away on its own. That said, there was one thing we could do to speed up her recovery: put her near a window. But weren't we supposed to keep the baby *out* of the sun, not in it? The answer is yes, but no. It turns out that sunlight, a natural source of vitamin D, is considered a safe and effective way of treating jaundice. When my parents came to visit us at the hospital, my dad wanted to hold Ashby and rock her in his arms. Would that be all right? Of course Da (his nickname deemed by his other grandkids) could hold his little sugar pie (yes, he already had a nickname for her). The only catch was, he had to sit next to the window. After a few minutes of rocking her in the sunlight, my dad turned to me and said, "Nan, I'm really hot." "Sorry, Dad. Ashby needs to stay in the window." Luckily, after a few more window treatments, Ashby's tiny bit of jaundice cleared right up.

No Need to Panic—Period

As the pediatrician was walking out the door after her initial visit with Ashby, she stuck her head back in and

said, "You know, Ashby may have a little bit of a period."
Fortunately, I had read that a newborn baby girl *might*
experience a little bit of bleeding from her vagina. Otherwise, I would have fainted. Before you feel anxious or
panicky, remember this occurrence is *totally* normal. The
light bleeding is caused by the withdrawal of the hormones your newborn was exposed to in the womb. The
bleeding usually lasts less than one day and is not painful for your baby. In fact, the bleeding is actually a good
sign. It means your baby has responded well to the drop in
hormone levels and her system is working properly. Who
knew!

What to Take with You When You Go Home

In my opinion, you should take everything the hospital gives you. *Everything*. Most hospitals will send you
home with a plastic tub filled with supplies. You will use
all of them.

※ Those amazing teeny tiny diapers (I didn't even know
they made diapers that small!)
※ The baby blankets that are the perfect size for swaddling
※ The little baby hat (The hospital-issued cap was the
only hat that didn't fall off Ashby's head.)
※ The hairbrush, which will help with cradle cap—
flaky, dry skin on your baby's head that kind of looks

like dandruff (Most often it appears in the first few months of your baby's life, and usually clears up on its own, in about six months.)

* The itty-bitty onesies, because they actually fit your baby

* The nasal aspirator, which will help expel leftover fluids (You might want to ask for an additional one of these. Trust me, the drugstore ones don't compare.)

* Hospital pacifiers (Something about them just works for newborns, and you'll never be able to keep track of just one.)

* And speaking of keeping track, ask the hospital to give you several "Infant Feeding Record" charts. You will use these while at the hospital to record when the baby has eaten, peed, and pooped, and you are supposed to write down these things for the first several weeks of your baby's life and report any unusual variations to your pediatrician. If you are breastfeeding, these charts help you keep track of when you nurse and on which breast (you have to treat them equally or they get jealous of each other—see pages 140–141).

* Even that plastic tub will come in handy (We used it to give Ashby her first several baths.)

Plus, don't be shy about *your* needs. The nurses were so sweet to send me home with a whole bag of maxi pads, several cans of analgesic spray (oh, I loved that stuff) for "that" area, and a couple of squirt bottles for cleansing. Take all of it.

Don't Forget the Keepsakes!

Most hospitals routinely make two copies of the baby's footprint, one for the hospital record and the other as a keepsake for you. So be sure to ask for your copy. Also: don't forget to save the baby's ID bracelet, yours, and your partner's, as well as the nameplate from the bassinet, and even the umbilical cord clip for your baby's scrapbook. You will be glad you saved all of that stuff!

Nonessentials: Fashionable Babywear

In addition to a gorgeous layette set for her to wear home, I'd brought multiple outfits to the hospital for Ashby. I remember thinking that she would need a new outfit for every day she was there—which was totally absurd. The hospital had brand-new, perfect little onesies for her. So not only did she not wear any of the clothes I packed for her, but when we put her in that newborn layette set, complete with hat, she was swimming in it (and remember, Ashby wasn't a small baby). I found this to be the case with most "newborn" clothes, most of which are marked zero to three months, so they have to be big enough to fit a three-month-old, too. So, for the first week, she lived in the hospital onesies, which we took home. My recommendation: Save those cute outfits for when family and friends come to visit. You never even see the outfit you put her in the day she goes home because the hospital wraps her up for you! So if you want to put her in something special, focus on the swaddling blanket.

Take Your Threshold Pictures

Just like that photo you have (mental or otherwise) of you and your mate crossing the threshold of your home for the first time as a married couple, be sure to ask a nurse to take a photo of you, your mate, and the baby exiting the hospital. Also, take one of you and your newly expanded family entering your house. Both are huge moments. Leaving the hospital with teeny tiny Ashby in my arms, thinking this fragile little being's life was now in my hands—where was the instruction manual?—was an unforgettable experience, and I love the photo we have of the three of us embarking on the adventure of a lifetime. And then that next photo (which we forgot to take and I regret to this day) says, you are now entering your new life together. Home sweet home has just gotten sweeter.

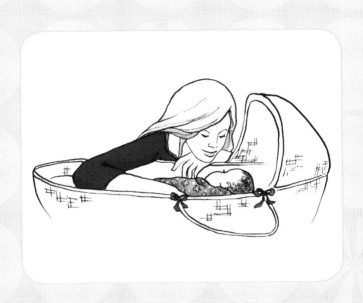

THE FIRST
WEEK HOME

Walking into my house for the first time with Ashby was one of the most surreal experiences of my life. I had just spent the last forty weeks being pregnant. It was hard to believe that this little human—whom I had planned for, meticulously eaten healthy meals for, and whose appearance I'd spent hours imagining—had actually arrived. And here she was, Ashby Grace, a miniature version of Keith and me staring right at Mama and Daddy with her big, beautiful baby eyes.

Keith had told me the feelings I would have after meeting her would be an overwhelming love like I had never felt before. I had always responded, "Yes, honey, of course it will be," as if he were telling me something that was common sense. But he was right, I didn't totally understand the gravity of the love I would feel *until* I held Ashby in my arms.

So many friends have said to me, "I'm so in love with my baby." I always thought that was an odd phrase. Wasn't being "in love" reserved for romance? But I totally get it now. You do fall in love. It's this massive, overpowering feeling that words cannot even begin to describe. All I wanted to do was hold her and care for her. I was giddy when she was awake and protective when she was asleep. I spent hours studying her hands and feet, counting her tiny fingers and toes. I was mesmerized by every little crevice and pudge. I was (and am) so utterly in love.

Big House, Small Baby

Ashby was so tiny, which made the house and everything in it feel huge. She was seven pounds, nine ounces at birth—a very healthy newborn size—and a little less when she left the hospital. (Babies typically lose a little weight after they're born. One theory as to why this happens is that they are born with extra fluid in their bodies that allows them to thrive on relatively little food until their mother's milk supply comes.) One thing you don't realize (unless you've been around a newborn recently) is that new babies are *teeny* teeny tiny. They're not the robust, pudgy babies we're used to seeing on TV and in movies (those babies are weeks—even months—older than newborns).

On top of that, Ashby seemed so delicate. Of course this made me feel anxious about everything I was doing. Did I take her out of the car seat the correct way? Was I holding her properly? Was I supporting her neck enough? But the good news was that we had arranged ahead of time to have a night nurse help us out in the evenings. So I knew that help was on the way and I'd soon settle into my new role.

Where to Find Help

Hiring someone to help me out with Ashby was something that had me in a complete panic. I knew it would be the most important hire I'd ever make—this person was going to help me care for my brand-new baby. This wasn't a decision I would make lightly. Since I had already decided to take three months' maternity leave, I needed only a night nurse in the beginning. Three months before my due date, I interviewed dozens of people through agencies, but none of them seemed right. Either they were too inexperienced, too young, too spacey, or too smokey. (Okay, who would show up for an interview for a job taking care of a baby smelling like a smokestack? Needless to say, that one did not get the job.) I was almost ready to give up when I turned to the hospital where I would give birth. During a tour, I asked around among staff if anyone knew of someone and an administrator told me about a wonderful nurse who had been at the hospital for twenty-three years, taking care of the newborns, and who did night nursing as well. It sounded too good to be true, but it was true and that's how wonderful Rita came into our lives. So now you know: The hospital is a great resource for childcare.

Many baby nurses do work on the side. The hospital will also know of a lot of retired nurses, many of whom do nanny or night nurse work. Who better to take care of your baby than a medical professional? I was sold!

The First Night Is the Toughest!

Rita, the highly recommended night nurse, was set to start on our first night back from the hospital. It was comforting to know she would be there. I had read books about taking care of a newborn during those first few weeks, but there I was, feeling like I knew *nothing*. We'd been home from the hospital for a couple of hours when I got the phone call: Rita had been in a car wreck on the way to our house. She wasn't hurt, but she sounded very rattled. She knew *I* was rattled (given it was my first night home with my new baby) and still wanted to come, but I couldn't ask her to do that. She could start the next day.

I hung up the phone and took a deep breath. *I can do this, right? Why am I worried? Women have been taking care of their newborns throughout history.* Needless to say, I didn't sleep a wink. Every ten minutes I had to make sure Ashby was still breathing. Then there were the harrowing few minutes when she broke free from her swaddle and was flailing about in her Moses basket—all three feet of it (the horror!). It was quite the cold plunge into parenting.

Meanwhile, Keith was as cool as a cucumber, snoring up a storm next to me. It was a long night, but in the end,

FULL *of* LIFE

it worked out just fine. Rita arrived the following evening, and I was so grateful for her help, even though I never wanted to leave Ashby's side. After several weeks, Rita would joke, "I don't know why you need me if you're going to wake up for every feeding. Just put some breast milk in a bottle so you can sleep." I didn't want to sleep, but I did need Rita. She was an encyclopedia of information!

Engorged Breasts

My milk had come in at the hospital, so by the time I brought Ashby home my breasts were beyond engorged. They looked more like bricks than breasts. It was excruciating. I had done some reading on the subject, so I knew that "engorgement" was considered a positive sign. It meant that I was producing milk to feed Ashby, which was great. It just felt as if I were producing enough milk to feed Ashby *and* the entire maternity ward at Cedars Sinai. On the first night that Rita was with us, she took one look at my breasts and said, "Honey, you've got to do something." And thank goodness, I did. By pumping a little and manually expressing some of the milk with my hand, I was able to soften my areola (the area around the nipple), which allowed Ashby to latch on with greater ease. Problem solved. Well, sort of. It took a few days for the initial engorgement to subside. But there were several things I was able to do to provide some relief. Here's what you can do if you find yourself in a similar circumstance:

- Keep your nursing bra on at all times. You're supposed to sleep in it every night! (Sorry, husbands. We still haven't gotten our sexy back yet.)
- Make sure to nurse as much as possible. (It'll help, and it's a great way to bond with your baby.)
- Use the cool breast gel packs on your nipples. They fit nicely into your nursing bra.
- Put a bag of frozen peas on your engorged breasts. It helps to ease the swelling.
- Don't forget to use lanolin nipple ointment to keep your nipples from cracking. (It isn't harmful to the baby.)
- Take a warm shower before you breastfeed, making sure to massage your breasts to soften the milk ducts. This will make nursing (and that initial latch-on) easier.

A SHOWER IN THE SHOWER

My sister, Karen, warned me that when I showered I might experience another kind of shower: a milk shower! That's right. The warm water helps your milk flow, and before you know it, you're springing a leak. Make that, shooting a leak! Mine even extended beyond the shower. So take note: line the floor outside the shower with towels before you get in, because when you come out, your milk may still be flowing. It took me a week's worth of milk showers and lots of cleaning up to learn this.

Pumping Power

I remember sitting cross-legged on the floor, surrounded by breast pump parts, feeling completely lost. There were containers, lids, and two "breastshields." Why did my breasts need shields? My Medela "Pump in Style" pump even boasted a "one-touch let-down button, designed for faster milk flow." Okay, now things were starting to sound scary. A let-down button? As I sat there, putting all the wrong pieces in all the wrong places, my night nurse burst out laughing. Thankfully, Rita showed me how to hook the whole thing up, where to attach the tubes, how to fit the breast shields into the suction cup thingy, and how best to place the device on my breast. My sweet mom so desperately wanted to help me, but electric breast pumps just didn't exist back in her day. They're modern mom machines, which you practically need a master's degree to operate.

I expected the whole pumping thing to be easy. It's not. And I'm not even going to try to explain how to do it here because I'll just confuse you. All I'll say is: get your breast pump before you have your baby, and enlist someone to show you how to use it. Try to buy your pump at a store that specializes in breastfeeding supplies—that way you can talk to an expert. *Or* talk to a lactation specialist weeks before you give birth, as I recommended; she can give you the 4-1-1.

Don't Even Think About It, Buddy

Let's be simple and straight, here. Your boobs are not your husband's. They're not even yours. They belong to the baby. So if you see your husband giving your breasts a lingering stare, as I caught Keith doing one night, just say no.

Around the Clock

Let me explain why your boobs belong to your baby. New babies eat *often*—roughly every two hours, if you're breastfeeding them. In the beginning you'll want to get in at least eight to twelve feedings a day, as this will not only keep your baby content but also establish your milk supply. For a newborn, you're supposed to nurse on demand. With Ashby, the nursing itself would take about forty-five minutes. Sometimes she would fall asleep while breastfeeding, and I'd have to wake her up by tickling her cheek, which added a few minutes here and there. After Ashby finished nursing on the first breast, there was the burping, the changing of positions, the changing of breasts, and, shortly thereafter, the changing of diapers. Then I would have to re-swaddle her to get her back to sleep, only to have her wake up again hungry in less than an hour. (This is where having an extra set of hands comes in handy—an eager grandmother, sister, or a night nurse will be of great help.) Here are a few tips I learned about feeding a newborn:

* Start with one breast. When that breast is completely emptied, burp your baby. Then offer him or her the second breast, but don't force the issue.
* Always keep track of which breast you started on, and then be sure to alternate every feeding.
* Remember those feeding logs I told you to bring home from the hospital? It's time to pull those out. You think you'll easily remember which breast you started on the last time, but trust me, you won't, because there are *so many* feedings.

CAUSE FOR EARLY DISMISSAL

If the baby pulls off before she finishes one breast, it probably means she needs to be burped right then (before you switch breasts). I learned this from Mama Z, who explained what was going on one day when, as I was sitting in the middle of the living room nursing Ashby (yes, once you start nursing, you quickly lose all sense of modesty) the baby suddenly popped off my breast. One quick pat and a loud belch later, and she was back in her boob groove.

Just Like Nursing, There Are Several Burping Positions

Who knew! Fortunately, I had my mom, Mama Z, and Rita to show me these different positions, and if

Ashby didn't burp with the first position, there was always the next one.

- **Over the shoulder.** Drape your baby over your shoulder with his or her stomach facing you and firmly pat his or her back.
- **Facedown.** Position your baby across your lap with his or her head resting on one leg and stomach across the other. Make sure baby's head is turned to the side. Support your baby with one hand and pat her with the other.
- **With baby sitting up.** Sit your baby on your lap and lean her chin into your hand, then rub gently upward and/or pat baby's back firmly.

Feather or Firm?

When I first burped Ashby I was beyond hesitant. I did the "feather burp," as Keith liked to call it. In other words, I couldn't get her to burp because I was barely patting her on the back. But Keith could get her to burp every time with his firm pats. So it's true what people say: babies are not as fragile as you think.

Happily-Ever-After Pains

Back at my baby shower, where my friends doled out their words of wisdom about the things that might happen during my pregnancy and after I had given birth, my friend Courtney wrote something in my scrapbook about "reverse contractions." I didn't understand what she meant until one day when I was sitting in the glider nursing Ashby. I was looking down at my beautiful little daughter, thinking, *this is like a fairytale,* when the fairy-tale moment was cut short by an excruciating cramp that felt like a menstrual cramp but far more intense. *Wait, I can't be getting my period,* I thought. (You don't usually menstruate when you're breastfeeding. Nursing acts as a natural suppressant, though there is postpartum bleeding.) I was sure something was wrong, so I called my doctor. He assured me that it was *nothing* to worry about. Those cramps (also known as "after pains") were the result of my uterus shrinking back to its pre-pregnancy size. (Apparently the pain becomes even more intense with each subsequent birth. Oh boy.) What had triggered those contractions? Nursing! When a woman breastfeeds, the hormone oxytocin is released, which stimulates your uterine muscles to start contracting. On the plus side, the pain, while surprising, is temporary and should last for only a week.

The Great Swaddling Debate

From the moment we brought Ashby home from the hospital, one of the hotly debated topics in our house was swaddling. If you are unfamiliar with the term, swaddling is a way to wrap a baby to make her feel as if she's back in the womb. When I was pregnant, all of my friends would speak glowingly about the power of swaddling. They sounded like members of some secret baby society ("if you swaddle, the baby *will* sleep"). And judging from the number of blankets I received at my baby shower, I knew there had to be some truth to it.

Rita could swaddle Ashby in 2.5 seconds, transforming her from a crying baby to a peacefully sleeping, neatly wrapped tortilla. Meanwhile, on the opposite end of the spectrum, my mom would always look at Ashby in her swaddle and shake her head. "That can't be right. The baby should be loose. Look at her. She wants to exercise her arms and legs." Back in my parents' day, swaddling wasn't en vogue. So, wondering what was the best for the baby, I asked Rita why she recommended swaddling. Rita explained that not only does it keep the baby warm, but the surrounding pressure seems to give most newborns a sense of security. (That sounds nice. I wouldn't mind a swaddle every now and then.) Now I just had to figure out how to do Rita's tortilla swaddle, which meant I needed a miracle.

MIRACLES DO HAPPEN

After sharing several stories of my poor swaddling skills with my friend Kim, she recommended I buy a "Miracle Blanket." And let me tell you, it truly was a miracle. It's made especially for swaddling-challenged folks like me. There are no snaps, no straps, no buttons . . . nothing to adjust, and one size fits all. And within a matter of minutes of purchasing it, I was a pro at swaddling, and Ashby had stopped fussing and was sleeping, once again, peacefully on her back. See, miracles *do* happen.

How to Relax Your Baby

One day I walked into the den and found Ashby asleep on her back on my dad's lap. My dad has really long legs, so he was the perfect cradle for a newborn. He used to brag that Ashby loved to hang out with him while he watched his ball games—it was *their* time. On one such occasion, I walked in and my dad called me over and said, "Come here. I've got something to show you." He looked so proud. He then demonstrated his trick: If he rubbed the space between Ashby's eyebrows, from her forehead to the bridge of her nose, she would close her eyes, relax, and eventually fall asleep. And sure enough, every time I used that trick, it worked!

We've Got Rhythm

Babies love rhythm. Even before they're born, babies are soothed by your steady walking. After they're born, babies love being rhythmically rocked. Ashby loved it when we held her and rocked her, shifting our weight from side to side at the same time, patting her in a steady beat. The minute I stopped, Ashby's eyes would open. (Think of rocking as your exercise time! Squeeze your buns as you rock back and forth.) Ashby's love of rhythm extended to music, too. There's a reason why there are so many lullaby CDs out there: they work! Ashby loved Baby Einstein Lullaby, Volume Two. It *had* to be Volume Two—she was a particular baby.

Water Baby

Another way to help your baby relax is to play the sound of falling water. I stumbled upon this technique by accident. One day, when Ashby was crying and Keith was on a business phone call, I walked outside with her. We have a fountain in our courtyard, and as soon as Ashby heard the sound of the water, she immediately grew calm and quiet. Evidently, babies love the sound of water. Perhaps, it has something to do with water being in the womb. If you don't have a fountain as a part of your home or garden, here are three great alternatives:

* A tiny fountain for the nursery.
* A nature CD that features water sounds.
* A stuffed animal that plays water or womb sounds. Lizzy, our future nanny, gave Ashby this cute little bear that played various water sounds (light rainfall, fountain, ocean rainstorm).

How to Get Your Baby to Take a Pacifier

I was on the fence about whether I wanted Ashby to use a pacifier. I had heard that they can lead to tooth problems and that it's hard to wean babies from them. But I was sold once Rita told me that pacifiers are strongly recommended to help prevent SIDS (sudden infant death syndrome) at bedtime. Plus, I read that when a baby sucks, it's a natural way for her to self-soothe. And sure enough, whenever Rita gave Ashby a pacifier, it would relax her. But when I would try to get her to take it, no dice. She'd spit it right out. My mom, having witnessed this, would tell me: "She's just like you. I could never get you to take a pacifier." After a few more failed attempts, I was almost ready to give up, when Rita shared this tip with me: She said, "Tap on the top of the binky while it's in her mouth, then pull it away from her ever so slightly. And, voilà. She'll start sucking the pacifier." It turns out that those simple moves help trigger a baby's natural sucking instinct. Later, I gave it a shot, and Ashby took the pacifier immediately.

Pacifier Particulars

* **Don't buy too many pacifiers—until you figure out which kind your baby likes.** I was given multiple kinds of pacifiers at my baby shower, each from a mom who swore that this was the one her baby loved. Once you know which one your baby likes, stock up.
* **Silicone vs. latex pacifiers.** I always chose silicone pacifiers because they were sturdier, cleaned up easier, and were harder for Ashby to bite through—and thus, sounded safer to me.

- **Be sure to replace pacifiers often.** You want to watch for signs of deterioration, because a worn or cracked nipple can pose a choking hazard for your baby. And when pacifiers get a sticky feel, it's time to toss them. Some manufacturers even recommend replacing pacifiers every four weeks.

- **Nix the necklace.** I chose never to use any kind of pacifier clip or string. I had heard too many warnings about their being potential strangulation hazards. My solution to pacifiers falling on the ground—because they will—was always to carry three or four extras in my purse.

- **Buy only one-piece pacifiers.** They reduce the chances of any pieces coming loose and choking a baby.

- **Buy pacifiers with a vented shield.** This helps prevent a rash around the mouth.

- **Always check for pacifier recalls.** You can do this at: www.cpsc.gov (U.S. Consumer Product Safety Commission).

Simply Sterile

When you first break open a package of breast pump parts, baby bottles, and pacifiers, always make sure to sterilize them before initial use, as they may contain chemical residue. I remember buying a pacifier from the store, taking it out of the package, and giving it to Ashby, thinking, "Hey, it's got to be clean. It's never been used before." Then, as I threw the packaging away, I noticed the bold letters: BE SURE TO STERILIZE BEFORE USING! *Oh no!* So, in addition to sterilizing everything *after* each use, be sure to sterilize brand-new items as well.

My motto became: when in doubt, boil it. There was a pot of boiling water on our stove all the time. I chose to do it the old-fashioned way, but there are many ways to sterilize: steamers, a dishwasher, microwavable bags. If you choose to boil as I did—that is, on your stovetop— there are a few things to know:

- ※ Prewash the items with soap and water. For bottles, you'll need a bottle brush, which is designed to clean inside the bottle (your regular scrubbie won't be able to reach inside). Some bottle brushes come with a nipple brush attached, and I recommend buying that all-in-one brush. Otherwise, you'll need a separate nipple brush to clean the inside of the nipples.
- ※ If you can't clean the bottle as soon as the baby finishes, let it soak in warm soapy water.
- ※ Once you're ready to boil the items, make sure you do it for at least five minutes.
- ※ Pull the items out with clean tongs and place them on a drying rack (there are even baby bottle racks designed for just this use).

* If it's a pacifier you're sterilizing, be sure to squeeze the remaining hot water out of the nipple. I used to use a paper towel to do it, that way I could ensure the pacifier stayed sterilized because it wasn't touched.

Say Cheese

Getting a baby to take a pacifier wasn't the only trick Rita had up her sleeve. One night I walked into the nursery and Ashby was smiling away at Rita. For a moment there, I was quite jealous. Rita teased me, "Oh, she doesn't smile like this for you?" She then told me that she could get Ashby to smile for her anytime, and she was right. Finally, she revealed her secret: She would tickle Ashby's chin, as if she were brushing off an invisible speck of dirt. And sure enough, a sweet smile would form across Ashby's face. Cheese!

Diaper Dos

Now that I had Ashby smiling, I wanted to keep her that way, which meant I had to figure out a way to make diaper changing a less traumatic experience. Ashby hated getting her diaper changed. She was such an even-tempered baby—until she needed a diaper change, at which point she'd cry the entire time, which made *me* almost cry the entire time. I finally learned, through trial and error, something very basic: When it comes to the diaper change, time is of the essence. You need to be speedy and efficient. Babies hate cold air, so make sure you have all of your supplies laid out, like an assembly line, ahead of time, to save time.

Diaper Duty Checklist

- Changing pad
- Clean diaper
- Gauze for wiping (Remember, for little girls, always wipe from front to back to avoid a urinary tract infection. I had to explain this one to Keith. Oh . . . *men*.)
- Container of warm water
- Diaper ointment with the cap off (FYI: You don't just put the ointment on *after* your baby has a rash. You put it on *every* time you change her, to *prevent* a rash.)

Diaper Do-Dos

You need to make sure your baby poops and pees a certain number of times every day. This, once again, is where those Infant Feeding Record charts come in handy. They have a place where you can chart wet and dirty diapers, which is important, because your baby's used diapers tell you if she is getting proper hydration/nutrition. Ask your pediatrician how many soiled diapers is correct for your baby. And note that the color and texture of your baby's bowel movements change pretty much daily the first week. They can range from tarlike black to a seedy yellow.

Visitors

Let's put this bluntly: You won't want visitors during the first week home. Heck, you won't want visitors for the first *many* weeks home. First of all, you'll be exhausted. Second, you won't have time to visit, as you'll be feeding your baby around the clock, and if you are nursing, you will most likely be leaving the room anyway. (Lack of modesty is usually only reserved for family members.) And third, a baby's immune system has not yet fully kicked in, so it is best to limit the germs to which they are exposed. So if you feel that you and your baby are not ready for visitors yet, have a nice excuse prepared when people express a desire to visit.

Back to Sleep!

Before Ashby was born, I knew how important a baby's sleep position was, and I went around quizzing everybody. "How do you put your baby to sleep? On her back? On her tummy? On her side?" Across the board, it seemed that people were not entirely sure. It wasn't until I asked my pediatrician that I got the definitive answer. The American Academy of Pediatrics says that on the back is the preferred sleep position for babies, as it provides the best protection against SIDS. This includes naps. So it's important for *everyone* caring for your baby to use the back sleep position. In addition, always make sure that your baby is placed on a firm sleep surface, which should be covered with a tight fitted sheet. You don't want your baby to be on or near loose bedding, as this also can contribute to SIDS.

Keep in mind, this is new advice, and until a few years ago, doctors and nurses had mothers place their infants on their stomachs to sleep. But research now shows that sleeping on the back lowers the risk of SIDS. So always remember: the back is best!

Additional Tips for Reducing the Risk of SIDS

* Clear the crib of squishy items—pillows, comforters, blankets, fluffy bumper pads, soft toys, sheepskin.
* Keep the baby's environment smoke-free.
* Use a safety-approved crib with a firm mattress and a snug fitted sheet.
* Educate grandparents and other caregivers on the latest SIDS safety recommendations.
* Don't allow the baby to get overheated with excessive clothing, bedding, or a room heater. (Rita told me about this one. The theory is that if the baby is too warm, he will think he's back in the womb and forget to breathe. Believe it or not, breathing is voluntary.)

Boob Food

When I found out I was pregnant, one of the first things my doctor did was to give me a list of foods I needed to avoid. No sushi. No unpasteurized cheeses. No raw eggs—which, I sadly learned, are in Caesar salad dressing. Darn it! So after I had the baby, I felt like I deserved a little indulgence. I mean, come on, I had been eating carefully for *forty weeks.*

So on one of our first nights home, I sat down for a meal of bruschetta (topped with tomatoes, garlic, and onion) and pizza. For dessert, I topped it off with several chocolate-covered strawberries, ice cream, and a *huge* glass of milk. I remember thinking, "Now that I'm breastfeeding, I should really drink some milk." Drink milk for making milk, right? Wrong! It turns out that the meal I had devoured contained practically every sinful food on the "do-not-eat" list for breastfeeding moms. In other words, unbeknownst to me, I had created the ultimate gas cocktail for my baby. That night, poor little Ashby was inconsolable, and I had no clue why.

Rita knew right away that Ashby was gassy, and asked me what I had eaten for dinner. I replied, "I ate *so* well. Tomatoes, onions, cheese, milk, strawberries—" She cut me off. "Oh, honey, you just ate every gassy food there is." I felt awful. No one had told me that there were foods I was supposed to avoid while nursing. Of course, I knew to limit my consumption of alcohol and caffeine. But beyond that, I had never heard anything about staying away from strawberries and broccoli. I mean, these were fruits and vegetables. Weren't they supposed to make Ashby grow big and strong—not cry in pain?

After doing some research, I learned that strongly flavored foods can sometimes cause a baby to become gassy and uncomfortable. The list of offenders often includes:

- ❋ Pizza
- ❋ Tomatoes
- ❋ Cauliflower
- ❋ Onions
- ❋ Anything dairy
- ❋ Broccoli
- ❋ Brussels sprouts
- ❋ Cabbage
- ❋ Beans
- ❋ Strawberries
- ❋ Chocolate

After hearing the list, I couldn't believe it. Everything I had eaten in that meal was on the list. My poor little baby! So why was this the first time I was hearing about this? Well, many folks consider altering one's diet to be the stuff of old wives' tales. That said, I was pretty confident that those foods affected Ashby, because she had never been colicky before. In fact, the only other time Ashby had had a gassy day was when I ate a cheese plate. (Again, dairy.) This is why I started to keep a breastfeeding food journal. That way, if Ashby ever seemed agitated or fussy after I nursed her, I could refer to my list and adjust my diet accordingly.

> ### YOU DON'T HAVE TO SAY GOOD-BYE
> ### TO MILK FOR GOOD
>
> Ashby's pediatrician told me that I could still have milk while I breastfed, which was good, because I still had a major craving for it. The catch was that it had to be lactose-free milk, which is readily available at grocery stores. But the good news is: stores carry lactose-free ice cream, too! One day my sweet father-in-law, Papa Z, came home from the grocery store with it, held it up, and said, "Look at what I found." It was *yummy.*

Postnatal Vitamins

After *The Great GAShby* incident, it really hit home that what *I* was eating, *she* was eating. Thankfully, one thing I'd been consuming that was helping her was my prenatal vitamins, which my doctor said I should continue doing, because I was nursing.

Strings Attached

As with all babies, when I brought Ashby home from the hospital she still had the remnants of her umbilical cord (i.e., the cord stump). Before we left, her pediatrician gave us a rundown on how to take care of it:

❋ While the umbilical cord area is healing, it's important to always keep the cord stump clean and dry. She told us to stick to sponge baths and to avoid tub baths until the stump fell off.

❊ The pediatrician also recommended not putting Ashby in tight-fitting clothes, as they can irritate the stump and cause infection, so we dressed Ashby in shirts, loose pants, and kimono-style shirts (which were great because we didn't have to pull them over her head).

❊ We also made sure to fold the front part of her diaper down, below the remainder of the umbilical cord.

The doctor told us we could expect Ashby's cord stump to fall off within ten to twenty-one days. And it did—but not all of it. Left in its place was a piece of red tissue that protruded from her belly button. I called Keith over and said, "Babe, what's that? I don't think that looks right." Keith agreed that it looked a little odd. But then, it didn't seem to bother Ashby, so we didn't totally panic. After a visit with the pediatrician, we learned that Ashby had what is known as an "umbilical granuloma." It is not serious and it isn't painful; it's just something that can form when the cord doesn't fully separate from the baby.

Phew, what a relief! So now what do we do? The doctor recommended that we make an appointment with a plastic surgeon. My eyes went wide. A plastic surgeon? I couldn't believe it. My daughter was only seven weeks old and she was already having her first visit with a plastic surgeon? Wow, we really are in Hollywood! The doctor laughed, then explained that the reason she wanted us to see a plastic surgeon was for him to confirm the granuloma. In the end, Ashby's plastic surgery procedure consisted of the surgeon holding a cotton swab on the tissue for about two seconds. The Q-tip had been dipped in silver nitrate, which burns the tissue off (the granuloma has no nerves, so it did not hurt Ashby at all). After the procedure, the tissue turned black then fell off. Now Ashby's belly button is all healed and she has an innie, just like her mama.

Taking Baby Steps

When I refer to taking baby steps, I'm not talking about Ashby, but myself. The best thing I can tell you is to be patient with yourself. When you're a new mother, there's a lot of information to learn. When we first brought Ashby home, there was a part of me that didn't totally trust my instincts. I didn't have my baby sea legs. Of course, everyone around me (Keith, my parents, my parent-in-laws) would always assure me that this was part of the learning curve, and I had to trust that it would get easier and that I would soon grow more comfortable. But still, I was terrified—which is crazy because I'm not normally a scaredy cat. And yet, I didn't even want Keith to leave the house to run errands. What if the baby needed to be changed? That was a two-person job! Well, not really. But I liked a spotter. I didn't feel that I knew what I was doing yet.

So unbeknownst to me, Keith came up with a plan. He would leave me alone at the house for ten minutes to "go run errands." Then he'd leave me alone for twenty minutes. Slowly, quietly, he was building up my confidence until, the next thing I knew, I was spending hours with Ashby, totally on my own. Ahh, Coach Keith really knows what he's doing! I promise you this: The confidence will come! It just takes a little time.

There's a learning curve to everything. Hey, it took me a while to get a handle on being pregnant, so of course it would take time to figure out the parenting thing. It's a whole new world for mother and daughter, but the best thing was that we were all a team!

Postpartum Elation

I'd heard so much about postpartum depression that after Ashby was born I kept checking myself for the warning signs. After reading several lists, I determined that I didn't have postpartum depression. But every time I held my brand-new baby, I did become very weepy. I would look down at her perfect little face and the next thing I knew, the tears were flowing. *But I'm beyond happy!* Turned out it was the sentimental, sweet, loving, bonding thoughts that brought on the tears.

One day Keith walked into the room while I was nursing Ashby and saw that I was crying. "Babe, what's wrong?" he asked. I looked up at him and said through tears, "Absolutely nothing." He asked me why I was crying. "I'm just so happy. I've never been happier in my whole entire life. I have a wonderful husband, two fabulous stepsons, and now my perfect Ashby. My life feels so blessed and complete with this amazing family," I said, still crying. It was at this point that my husband gave me my diagnosis. (I didn't need to call my doctor for this one.) Keith said, "Babe, what you have is *postpartum elation*." And he couldn't have been more right.

There was just something about staring down at my little girl and realizing the profound feeling of love I had for her. It made me think about my own mother, who had always made us feel so loved, but it was at this particular point that I realized the immense depth of her love for my sister and me. And here I was, now a mother myself. I guess that's why they call it the circle of life.

Concluding Note: Yes, you go through a bunch of unexpected, often embarrassing, sometimes scary things when you have a baby. But in the end, it's all worth it, because you get the best gift anyone could ever possibly receive!

ACKNOWLEDGMENTS

To Jen Bergstrom, Emily Westlake, Jennifer Robinson, and all at Simon Spotlight Entertainment, thanks for making the work on this book an amazingly enjoyable, professional, and overall incredible experience!

To Jessica, thanks for your way with words, your sense of humor, for putting up with my unpredictable schedule, and for jumping up and down with me in excitement when Ashby said "apple" for the first time!

To Peter, thanks for helping make this book happen and for truly caring as my manager and my friend.

To Lizzy and Julie, thanks for being such good and honest people that I trust you with my most precious daughter. Lizzy, thanks for letting me steal you away from *Access Hollywood* and alleviating my panic in finding a wonderful person to become our nanny. And Julie, thanks for immediately loving Ashby as you have my family all these years. And to both of you, I appreciate your support and extra hours while writing this book.

To my ob-gyn, whose privacy I will maintain. Thanks

for always being so calm, sincere, reassuring, and answering my hundreds of questions.

To Dr. Sloninsky, thanks for being such a compassionate pediatrician and for always being just a phone call away.

To Rob, Claudia, and Linda, thanks for your genuine happiness when you found out I was pregnant and for your support of this book.

To my Coastal Academy girlfriends, thanks for your lifelong, dear, and true friendship and for all your pregnancy advice.

To Joe S., Joe P., Lauren, and Aimee, thank you for your assistance and loyalty always. I wouldn't have had time for this book had you not been helping me with so many things.

To Mark, thanks for jumping right in and handling all the last-minute details.

To Karen, Nicole, Courtney, and Shaun, thanks for your friendship and for the beautiful baby showers you threw me with the fun games, which helped me realize the need for this book.

To Rita, thanks for all the talks while I was nursing, for your wonderful way with babies, and for teaching me so much about newborns.

To Mama Z and Papa Z, thanks for being such incredible parents-in-law and grandparents, and for your love and your words of wisdom during my pregnancy and after. Thanks for the million and one things you do to help us, like Mama Z's delicious cooking, which kept us all fed while I was writing, and Papa Z's lattes, which helped get me through editing the last chapters at crunch time.

To my sister, Karen, thanks for being a great big sis and allowing me to always laugh and cry with you when needed. Thanks for calling me every few days to see if I had a positive pregnancy stick. And thanks for reassuring me at every turn.

To my dad, thanks for being the most amazing father and "Da" to Ashby. Thanks for being such a wonderful husband to Mom. Your loving relationship with Mom has been an inspiration to me and Keith.

To my stepsons, Tyler and Carson, I am so blessed to have you both in my life. Thank you for being such amazing boys and great big brothers to Ashby. You are rock stars to her!

And to my husband and best friend, Keith, where do I begin?! Thanks for allowing me to share our story and for putting up with all those late-night writing sessions. You are the most incredible father, husband, and friend. I feel so lucky and blessed you are mine, and I fall more in love with you every day. You brought Carson and Tyler into my life and we created Ashby together and, for that, I thank you for making me full of life!

NOTES

Printed in the United States
By Bookmasters